Praise for *The Breathable Body*

"This loving book comes from the heart of love of a daring explorer of the mysteries of the body. Open anywhere and be reminded how delicious it can be to simply take a breath."

— **Lorin Roche, Ph.D.**, author of *The Radiance Sutras: 112 Gateways to the Yoga of Wonder and Delight* and *Meditation Made Easy*

"If I had to choose among the many books on breath and breathing, The Breathable Body *is without question the one I would choose. While clarifying the anatomy, physiology, chemistry, and mechanics of breathing, Litman shows how breathing is a whole-body phenomenon of our dynamic, fluid organism. His depth and breadth of knowledge are present in each explanation and exploration, and if you are one of the millions suffering from a breathing, sleep, or anxiety disorder, chances are the information you need is in this book."*

— **Don St John, Ph.D.**, author of *Healing the Wounds of Childhood and Culture: An Adventure of a Lifetime*

"Robert Litman shows how you can change your health, your mood, and your connection to all of life by changing how you breathe. Whether you struggle with breathing, need effective strategies for self-regulation, or want to more fully enjoy the pleasures of being alive, this book will provide insight and solutions to some surprisingly common health conditions. The Breathable Body *is an essential tool for good health!"*

— **Sharon Weil**, Registered Somatic Movement Educator, author of *ChangeAbility: How Artists, Activists and Awakeners Navigate Change*

"Litman draws on more than three decades of experience working with clients to bring together a resource accessible to everyone. What sets The Breathable Body *apart is the connection it highlights between body and breath, and how breathing and movement are linked. Your doctor may not have told you about the benefits of breathing re-education.* The Breathable Body *does just that! If you breathe, this book is for you."*

— **Patrick McKeown**, Director of Education and Training at Buteyko Clinic International and author of *The Oxygen Advantage*

"Robert provides a well-crafted paeon to the sacred and healing act of breathing; it is anatomy as poetry, required reading for anyone interested in the healing aspects of conscious breathing."

— **Karen M Gardner**, Ph.D. in Information Science, UC Berkeley

"Combining memoir, breathing therapy, and inquiry into the dynamic movement of body and mind, The Breathable Body *offers deep insights and practical instructions on every page. This is a highly relatable book you'll return to again and again for sagely advice."*

— **Matteo Pistono**, author of *Meditation: Coming to Know Your Mind* and *In the Shadow of the Buddha*

"Robert delivers a message in The Breathable Body *that has the potential to not only improve your health but also enhance the quality of your life. He has managed to bridge the gap between cognitive understanding of the scientific knowledge of breathing processes while guiding his readers into an immediate somatic participation with the material. This book offers a transmission of intimate presence with oneself and a reminder that the sacred resides in the present moment."*

— **Gael Rosewood**, Continuum teacher, certified Rolfer, and CE teacher and mentor for both modalities

"Conscious breathing has become a psychospiritual and energy-medicine meme, popularized in bodywork, yoga, and meditation circles to a degree that makes breathing so hyperconsciously conscious that it becomes even more unconscious. It *takes a breath practitioner who has been through its many layers of morphogenesis, phenomenology, dynamic function, micromovement, and personal unlayering to teach you how to make your breathing more endurably conscious. Robert Litman is a true breath healer, explorer, and teacher."*

— **Richard Grossinger**, author of *Bottoming Out the Universe* and *Dreamtimes and Thoughtforms*

"Robert draws you into the world of breath like nothing I've read before! Whether you are looking for help for an ailment or want to enrich your life through breath, this book—steeped with rich resources to expand and explore breathing—is for you."

— **Bobbie Ellis**, Continuum teacher and 500+ Experienced Registered Yoga Teacher

"Robert Litman takes us on a psychological journey, leading us through his own history with breathing and the metaphor for life that it has come to hold for him. Based on his hard-won wisdom, he guides us in practical ways that have helped so many—how to bring conscious breathing meaningfully into our lives."

— **Peter M. Litchfield**, President, Graduate School of Behavioral Health Sciences, lecturer in respiratory psychophysiology, self-regulation science, and many other subjects

"Breath spirals, listens, touches us on the inside, responds to kindness, tenderness, compassion, and gentleness, whispering its wildness into us. Others teach the science of breath, measuring and counting. Robert transmits the art and flow, letting breath lead us into the unknown. The Breathable Body *offers a glimpse into the author's love affair with breath, a quiet transmission into the most profound relationship we have. What a treasure this book is!"*

— **Roxanne Rhodes**, Certified Yoga Instructor, Trager practitioner, and massage therapist

THE
BREATHABLE
BODY

Hay House Titles of Related Interest

YOU CAN HEAL YOUR LIFE, the movie,
starring Louise Hay & Friends
(available as an online streaming video)
www.hayhouse.com/louise-movie

THE SHIFT, the movie,
starring Dr. Wayne W. Dyer
(available as an online streaming video)
www.hayhouse.com/the-shift-movie

***

MEDITATION MADE EASY: Coming to Know Your Mind,
by Matteo Pistono

FOCUS: Bringing Time, Energy, and Money into Flow,
by Pedram Shojai, O.M.D.

A FIERCE HEART: Finding Strength, Courage, and Wisdom
in Any Moment, by Spring Washam

THE POWER OF VITAL FORCE: Fuel Your Energy,
Purpose, and Performance with Ancient Secrets
of Breath and Meditation, by Rajshree Patel

All of the above are available at your local bookstore,
or may be ordered by visiting:

Hay House USA: www.hayhouse.com®
Hay House Australia: www.hayhouse.com.au
Hay House UK: www.hayhouse.co.uk
Hay House India: www.hayhouse.co.in

THE BREATHABLE BODY

TRANSFORMING YOUR WORLD AND YOUR LIFE, ONE BREATH AT A TIME

ROBERT LITMAN

HAY HOUSE, INC.
Carlsbad, California • New York City
London • Sydney • New Delhi

Copyright © 2023 by Robert Litman

Published in the United States by: Hay House, Inc.: www.hayhouse.com®
Published in Australia by: Hay House Australia Pty. Ltd.: www.hayhouse.com.au
Published in the United Kingdom by: Hay House UK, Ltd.: www.hayhouse.co.uk
Published in India by: Hay House Publishers India: www.hayhouse.co.in

Cover design: Scott Breidenthal • *Interior design:* Karim J. Garcia
Indexer: Joan Shapiro • *Illustrations:* Jill Elizabeth Zimmermann

All rights reserved. No part of this book may be reproduced by any mechanical, photographic, or electronic process, or in the form of a phonographic recording; nor may it be stored in a retrieval system, transmitted, or otherwise be copied for public or private use—other than for "fair use" as brief quotations embodied in articles and reviews—without prior written permission of the publisher.

The author of this book does not dispense medical advice or prescribe the use of any technique as a form of treatment for physical, emotional, or medical problems without the advice of a physician, either directly or indirectly. The intent of the author is only to offer information of a general nature to help you in your quest for emotional, physical, and spiritual well-being. In the event you use any of the information in this book for yourself, the author and the publisher assume no responsibility for your actions.

Cataloging-in-Publication Data is on file at the Library of Congress

Tradepaper ISBN: 978-1-4019-6891-5
E-book ISBN: 978-1-4019-6892-2
Audiobook ISBN: 978-1-4019-6893-9

10 9 8 7 6 5 4 3 2 1

1st edition, May 2023

Printed in the United States of America

FOR THE LOVE OF BREATH

Oh, for the love of breath that travels tenderly
through the interior of my body
like a breeze that stirs the leaves of a tree.
Oh, for the love of breath that delivers me
into an intimate relationship with my experience,
inviting the body and breath to move as one.
Oh, for the love of breath that is consciously revealing
the many possible pleasures
that are embedded in the movement of breath:
kindness, softness, flow, aliveness, ease, and love.
Oh, for the love of breath that reminds me to be grateful
for the gift of life, birthing me again and again with each new breath.

This book is dedicated to *breath*.
Breath never lies to me and always holds me accountable.
I bow in gratitude for its invitations to rediscover
the heart of innocence and beauty.

TEXT PERMISSIONS

Excerpt taken from the *Complete Jewish Bible* by David H. Stern. Copyright © 1998. All rights reserved. Used by permission of Messianic Jewish Publishers, 6120 Day Long Lane, Clarksville, MD 21029. www.messianicjewish.net.

Emilie Conrad, excerpt from "Continuum Movement" in *New Dimensions in Body Psychotherapy*, edited by Nick Totton (Open University Press, 2005). Reprinted by permission. Excerpt from "Continuum Movement" in *USA Body Psychotherapy Journal*, vol. 4, no. 1 (2005): 29. Copyright © 2005 United States Association for Body Psychotherapy. Reprinted with permission.

Clarissa Pinkola Estés, excerpt from *Women Who Run with Wolves: Myths and Stories of the Wild Woman Archetype*. Copyright © 1996 by Clarissa Pinkola Estés. Used by permission of Penguin Random House LLC. All rights reserved.

Diana Farid, excerpt from *When You Breathe*, illustrated by Billy Renkl. Text copyright © 2020 by Diana Farid. Used by permission of Cameron + Company, an imprint of ABRAMS, New York. All rights reserved.

Thich Nhat Hanh, excerpt from *Stepping into Freedom: An Introduction to Buddhist Monastic Training, Second Edition*, translated by Sister Annabel Laity. Copyright © 2021 by Plum Village Community of Engaged Buddhism, Inc. Reprinted with the permission of Parallax Press.

Matt Licata, excerpts from *A Healing Space: Befriending Ourselves in Difficult Times*. Copyright © 2020 by Matt Licata. Used with permission of the publisher, Sounds True, Inc.

Amit Ray, excerpt from *Om Chanting and Meditation: A Way to Health and Happiness* (Inner Light Publishers, 2010). Reprinted with permission.

Lorin Roche, excerpts from *The Radiance Sutras: 112 Gateways to the Yoga of Wonder and Delight*. Copyright © 2014 by Lorin Roche. Used with permission of the publisher, Sounds True, Inc.

David Suzuki, excerpt from *The Sacred Balance: Discovering Our Place in Nature*. Copyright © 2007 by David Suzuki. Reprinted with the permission of Greystone Books.

Morihei Ueshiba, excerpt from *The Art of Peace: Teachings of the Founder of Aikido*, by Morihei Ueshiba, translated © 2002 by John Stevens. Reprinted by arrangement with The Permissions Company, LLC on behalf of Shambhala Publications Inc., Boulder, Colorado, shambhala.com.

U.S. Sports Camps, excerpt from "Basketball Tip: How to Master the Jump Shot." Copyright © U.S. Sports Camps. Reprinted with permission.

From Rabbi Arthur Waskow, "Three Outcries and a Prayer," read during Shabbat Services June 18, 2022 on the Washington Mall during the Poor People's Campaign. For more about "interbreathing," see Arthur Waskow, *Dancing in God's Earthquake* (Maryknoll, NY: Orbis Books, 2020).

FIGURE PERMISSIONS

Line drawings © Jill Elizabeth Zimmermann, www.JilleZ.com, with the exception of the following:

Line drawing of figure in profile breathing through nose at the beginning of each Exploration: Yulia Sutyagina.

Photo of mother and son showing affection: Creatas / Getty Images

Photo of Sanya Richards: Reuters / Alamy Stock Photo.

Figures on pages 65 and 66 from *The Science of Breath: A Practical Guide*, by Swami Rama, Rudolph Ballentine MD, and Alan Hymes MD. Copyright © 1979, 1998 by The Himalayan International Institute of Yoga Science and Philosophy of the USA. Reprinted with the permission of the Himalayan Institute, Honesdale, Pennsylvania.

"Interview Checklist": Copyright © 2014 by Peter M. Litchfield, Ph.D. and Sandra Reamer MFA. Reprinted with permission.

J'inspire, J'expire

In many of the world's creation myths, God infuses breath into the first human and thus creates life. The first chapter of the Yukti Verses of the Radiance Sutras recounts a conversation between Shiva, the divine masculine ("The One Who Is Intimate to All Beings"), and Shakti, the divine feminine ("The Energy of Creation and Destruction").

Shakti asks Shiva,
How does spirit manifest into [human] form?

The One Who Is Intimate to All Beings replies,
Beloved, your questions require the answers that come
Through direct living experience.

The way of experience begins with a breath,
Such as the breath you are breathing now.
Awakening into luminous reality
May dawn in the momentary throb
Between any two breaths.

Exhaling, breath is released and flows out,
There is a pulse as it turns to flow in.
In that turn, you are empty.
Enter that emptiness as the source of all life.

Inhaling, breath flows in, filling, nourishing.
Just as it turns to flow out,
There is a flash of pure joy—
Life is renewed.[1]

How, then, shall we live, within a life span of breaths?

CONTENTS

FOREWORD

When Robert Litman began telling the world about breathing more than three decades ago, many people thought: "But breathing is natural. Why bother fixing it?"

In the years since, breathing has become a global movement. Vast numbers of people now understand and apply breathing techniques to improve stress levels, asthma, high blood pressure, breathing-disordered sleep, and states of mind. These breathing techniques are supported by large-scale studies and indisputable evidence.

This movement is all about *Breathing for the People*. Breathing is an amazing tool, one that's available on demand, free and accessible to everyone, and all that's needed is a deeper understanding of the breath and how to use it to your benefit. *The Breathable Body* teaches exactly that.

The teachings in this book will allow you to:

- Activate your body's relaxation response in as little as 30 seconds

- Decongest your nose

- Increase the temperature of your hands and feet within three to four minutes

- Lower high blood pressure

- Improve sleep and wake up feeling more refreshed and alert

- Reduce coughing and wheezing by 50 percent within a couple of weeks

- Boost your immune system

- And much more

To fully understand the breath, a few myths need to be debunked:

Myth # 1: Taking a deep breath

The word *deep* is commonly equated with *big;* and most people, when instructed to take a deep breath, respond by inhaling a large volume of air into their lungs. While taking a big breath might feel good in the short term, it reduces oxygen delivery to the brain and body; and if done consistently, it can contribute to stress, anxiety, and several health complications.

Myth # 2: It doesn't matter whether you breathe through your nose or your mouth

You might think I'm nitpicking here; however this is a major issue with serious consequences. Any child or adult who persistently breathes through an open mouth is likely to experience higher stress, poorer sleep quality, dental health issues, and lower energy, immunity, and resiliency.

Myth # 3: The more air you breathe, the better

With breathing, less is more. Unfortunately, breathing more air is encouraged in many breathwork practices. Audible breathing takes place as the instructor encourages participants to inhale as much oxygen and exhale as much carbon dioxide as they can. This way of breathing reduces carbon dioxide in your system, which contrary to popular belief, is not just a waste gas. Danish physiologist Christian Bohr discovered more than a century ago that carbon dioxide in the blood facilitates the transmission of oxygen from the blood to the tissues and organs.

Myth # 4: Awareness is the key for anxiety

Breathing changes in response to stress, and stress levels change in response to breathing. Breathing through an open mouth, over-breathing, and frequent sighing all feed into anxiety, and studies show that 75 percent of those who are anxious have poor breathing patterns. Because of this, bringing awareness to the breath is often recommended to help manage anxiety. However, central features of anxiety include a racing mind, an inability to stop thinking, and emotional turmoil. Expecting a person to be mindful and place their attention on their breath in these moments isn't exactly realistic. They'd be much more likely to benefit from practicing the simple breathing exercises explained in this book in everyday life. Doing so would change their physiology and regulate their nervous system so that they feel less stress in the first place.

Closing Thoughts

In *The Breathable Body*, Robert Litman brings together three-and-a-half decades of research and experience working with body and breath. This is a tremendous resource, as body and breath are intertwined. If one is off, the other is off, too. One little-known example is the connection between lower back pain and the breath. Faulty breathing compromises movement and the stabilization of the spine, and 50 percent of people with lower back pain have faulty breathing. In order to reverse lower back pain, therefore, faulty breathing patterns must be addressed. Robert's book uncovers this link and so many more!

I could spend hours discussing the benefits of applying scientifically based breathing exercises, but you are not here to listen to me. You are in good hands with Robert Litman's wonderful book, *The Breathable Body*. Enjoy the journey.

Patrick McKeown
author of *The Oxygen Advantage* and *The Breathing Cure*

ACKNOWLEDGMENTS

I would like to begin by thanking the many people who contributed to the lifesaving efforts needed at my birth: my father, who traveled to hospitals throughout New York City to obtain blood for the transfusions that kept me alive; the taxi drivers who drove him around; those who donated the blood that became my life force; and the doctors who were just learning about Rh-incompatible babies and how to keep them alive. This was the beginning of my journey into breathing, and my gratitude knows no bounds.

Thanks to my wife, Nell Luce, who inspires me with her confidence, honesty, beauty, fierceness, and love. And to my children, Jodi, Steve, Kelly, and stepdaughter, Meghan, who remind me of the power of love.

I thank my teachers in breath: Dr. Konstantin Buteyko, Jennifer Stark, Sandra Reamer, and Peter Litchfield. My teachers in structural integration: Annie Duggan and Janie French. My mentors in movement: Emilie Conrad, who opened the door for self-exploration through Continuum, which she created, and who became my best friend and collaborator for 18 years; Susan Harper of Continuum Montage, who deepened my access to my emotional landscape through her workshops, teachings, and friendship; and Continuum teachers and students everywhere. Thanks to Gael Rosewood, co-creator of the Continuum Wellsprings program after Emilie's death, dear friend for over 30 years and co-teacher for too many years to count. Gael's emotional intelligence, precision, and honesty continue to enhance my teaching and my capacity to listen to the needs of others. Thanks to Bobbie

Ellis, who has been my steadfast and loving teaching partner, creating depth, poetry, and intelligence in our sharing of Continuum for the benefit of our students and in my work as a writer. Thanks to my Wednesday-morning Continuum Dive pod: Bonnie Gintis, Laura Lawton, Linda Rabin, Robin Becker, Sabine Mead, Kim Brodey, Cory Blake, Suzanne Wright Crain, Rebecca Lawson, and Ellen Cohen, who provided connection, love, and authenticity to the process of Continuum during the pandemic, when our only contact was through Zoom. Special thanks to Sharon Weil, who made my study of Continuum possible with her love and friendship and enriched my life in innumerable ways that will forever have my deepest gratitude. And to Carole Burstein, who transformed my understanding of the psyche and personal behavior, adding immeasurably to my life and my teaching. And a big thank you to Barbara C. of the UK for providing financial assistance that allowed me to study and practice Buteyko Breathing Education.

I thank Roxanne Rhodes, who read pages and pages of this manuscript and offered thoughtful and insightful feedback. Thank you, Jill Elizabeth Zimmerman, for your beautiful work on the illustrations. Sincere thanks to my editors at Hay House, Matteo Pistono and Sally Mason-Swaab, who stood by me through the lengthy process of creating audio courses and meditations and the book you hold in your hands; and to my editor, friend, and occasional student Arnie Kotler, whose constancy allowed me to forge on even in moments of doubt. I thank the many other colleagues, students, clients, and friends who have helped in countless ways, giving me the love and support I needed to bring this vision into reality. As the book was nearing completion, I reached out to many of you for help financially so I could give my full attention to writing and editing. A special thanks to everyone who generously donated to help this book come to fruition. I could not have done it without you.

And finally, I thank breath itself. I have benefited more than words can convey by learning to trust breath's inherent intelligence, listen to the wide range of its messages, and accept its invitation to inquire deeply in support of wellness and in support of life itself.

MY JOURNEY WITH BREATH: AN INTRODUCTION

Breath flows
Into this body
As a nectar of the gods.
Every breath is a whisper
Of the Goddess.

— RADIANCE SUTRAS[1]

Everybody breathes. When we're breathing well, air enters our body with no manipulation on our part, and as breathing moves unrestricted, breath and body become attuned, and we abide in harmony within—making wise choices that enhance wellness. We are a part of a global community breathing ourselves into life.

We may only notice our breathing only when it becomes difficult to breathe and we experience symptoms like allergies, asthma, brain fog, dizziness, chronic obstructive pulmonary disease (COPD), emphysema, sleep apnea, snoring, breathlessness or shortness of breath, constantly needing to take a deep breath, exercise-induced asthma (a narrowing of the airways in the lungs triggered by strenuous exercise), chronic cough, and fatigue. But we don't need to wait until we have one of these disorders to become mindful of our breathing. We can tune in to our breathing right now and, through noticing its behavior, learn more about ourselves.

The term *breathable body* came to me during a meditation, and over time I've come to understand it to mean *"breathing with our whole body"*—in sync with our metabolic activity and having resilience in the face of stress, trauma, and pollutants. Having a body that breathes in harmony with its needs is a foundation stone for good health, stronger immunity, and a more satisfying life. But over the course of a lifetime, in response to real and perceived dangers, through habits and compensations, we begin to breathe in ways that no longer support optimal health.

I've studied my own and others' breathing and offered breathing education classes and workshops for almost 40 years. Many breathing therapies help us calm our nervous systems, increase vagal tone, and enhance athletic performance, and they can be a doorway to personal and spiritual growth. Of these, the modalities I rely on the most are Continuum and Buteyko Breathing Education.

Continuum was created by Emilie Conrad over 55 years ago to explore the fluid nature of the body. By connecting with and becoming aware of our fluid nature using breath, sound, and micro (very small) wave movements, she helped bring into awareness the subtle and profound intelligence of our bodies. Emilie described her work as "the mind falling back in love with the body."

Buteyko Breathing was developed in the 1950s by Konstantin Buteyko, a Ukrainian physician, who observed that the larger the volume of air people took to breathe, the sicker they became, and that training people to use less air led to the reduction or elimination of many symptoms and the restoration of health.

Breathing is a sacred act. It starts with an inhale, a moment of creation, and the rollover from inhale to exhale continues our journey through the cycle of breathing. All that we experience during a single round of breath comes to rest at the end of the exhale, as we wait for the next inhale and a new sequence to begin.

Each breath builds on the biological and emotional experiences of all preceding breaths. Breath's ultimate purpose is to nourish our aliveness, support movement, and create a field in which we can flourish. We breathe to awaken and sustain life.

Every day I ask my breath, *What can I learn from you today? What do I need to discover or remember?* Whenever I ask breath what it has to teach me, I always receive an answer. Breath communicates through sensation. So after asking what I need to learn, I observe the *feeling* and *movement* of the next breath—the temperature, texture, length, pace, rhythm, and steadiness—and each time I discover something new, something that sparks my creativity and love of beauty, or I'm reminded of something I've been overlooking that is calling for my attention.

Breath's responses to my questions are sometimes simple, like *Remember to use the back of your lungs when you breathe,* or *If you place your shoulders back and down, breathing will be easier.* At other times, breath's answers push me to the depths of my insecurities, revealing long-forgotten memories I've been holding in my body's tissues that are, at last, ready to be seen, felt, understood, and released. And sometimes breath's answer is simply to open my eyes and enjoy the world and those around me. I stay in conversation with my breathable body all day long, inspired by the words of activist and scholar Angela Davis: "You have to act as if it were possible to radically transform the world. And you have to do it all the time."

As I learned to be intimate with my own breathable body, I came out of the deep freeze of childhood trauma and into a fulfilling life with myself and others. After a lifetime of struggles with my own breathing, I do all I can now to support others' access to the power of breath and movement. And of all the things I've learned from breath, foremost among them is the importance of breathing in ways that are nourishing and sustaining. Our *breathable body* can be an intimate friend as we discover how to activate our innate inner intelligence and discern what breath is trying to tell us about ourselves. Gaining a felt sense of the rhythms and textures of breathing and their potential to provide life-sustaining nourishment can change our world. Everything else follows.

* * *

As a child, I withdrew into a veil of self-protection, a process that began in the womb. I was the fifth pregnancy of my soon-to-be parents. None of the other babies survived, and my parents were advised not to try again. My mother's blood was Rh-negative. I'm Rh-positive (as were my siblings), so my mother's body produced antibodies to attack our red blood cells, creating the risk for hemolytic disease of the newborn (HDN), which can cause brain damage or death in a fetus or newborn. My mother's antibodies were trying to destroy these cellular invaders in her womb, which meant *me*. Today a simple injection can stop that destructive process, but in 1944, when I was born, there wasn't much information about how to treat these kinds of pregnancies. So, from the moment of my conception, I had to fight for my life. Fortunately, a blood specialist recommended that immediately after my birth, my blood be replaced with blood that didn't have my mother's antibodies. So I stayed in the hospital for six weeks—without the consistent presence of a parent—while I received transfusions of lifesaving blood.

My father took taxis to hospitals all over New York City to pick up the blood for me, a hero's journey to keep his only surviving child alive. After my parents' fear, anguish, and disappointment arising from losing four babies, I was a gift they deeply cherished. But their fear prevailed, and they were rarely able to express their cherishing in a clear and straightforward way.

Both my parents were alcoholic. Over and over as I was growing up, my father would say to me, "You're worthless. You'll never amount to anything." My mother would be drinking by 11 A.M., following a night of drinking, and she'd say things like, "You're so handsome, the girls will be chasing you." The thought of being chased terrified me, and then *she* would chase me, and in her drunken state, she'd kiss me inappropriately. I felt revulsion and, beneath that, a pain still lives in my heart.

As babies and young children, we have highly sensitive nervous systems. We learn about the world and our environment through our senses. We touch, smell, see, hear, and taste the world, going toward what feels nourishing and away from what feels threatening. I probably began developing "armor"—layers of self-protection separating myself from the environment around me—in utero. And by the time I was 13, and probably earlier, I developed cough-variant asthma. Rather than wheeze like most asthmatics, I coughed myself into breathlessness. It was the 1950s, and my father told me over and over, "There's nothing wrong with you. Get your head on straight and you'll be able to breathe." So, we never went to see a doctor. I know now that asthma can be part of an array of PTSD symptoms.

I now also know that my parents did cherish me. When I was a grown man and my father was dying, he finally shared his heart. And I understand my mother's abusive behavior as her distorted way of expressing love. But as a child, I felt as though danger was everywhere, and I knew that my life was out of balance and I could die from not being able to take the next breath.

At school, my grades were poor, and my report cards always said I wasn't living up to my potential. But there was one bright light. I loved biology and was always able to take refuge in science classrooms and labs. The field of biology made sense to me. It was basic and honest, traits I revere, and this interest has stayed with me all my life and guided me to the recovery I needed to be empathetic—truly human.

I managed to get accepted into the University of Miami, Florida, which at the time was considered a party school. I only discovered when I got there that it also has one of the best marine biology programs in the country, so as a first-year student, I majored in marine biology. But the marine biology department was far from the main campus, where I had my other classes, and far from my dorm; there was no way to make it work. So I changed majors.

I met my first wife during our junior year, and we got married right out of college. We moved to New York, where I got a job as a junior account executive in a fashion-industry advertising agency.

But when my bosses asked me to bring in new accounts, I just couldn't. I was too afraid to put myself in that position, and I was laid off.

My wife was skilled at drawing me out. She was able to break through my protective barriers, and I expressed feelings I didn't know I had. We had two children, Jodi and Steve, both lights of my life. With them I could open my heart and pour out love long suppressed. But these states of joy and vulnerability were fragile. I could feel them in the safety of our home, but when I went out in the world, I would rebuild the armor. Then when I got back home, it was difficult to soften again. It took long, intimate conversations to melt me back to where my wife and family could feel my heart, a pattern that repeated day after day. I wanted the openness I felt with my family, but it wasn't available to me outside the house.

My wife and daughter had severe asthma. So, after I got fired from my position in New York, we moved to Arizona for cleaner, warmer air, and I began to work for an advertising agency in Tucson. After that and a series of other jobs, I began delivering newspapers from midnight till 6 A.M. seven days a week, driving a hundred miles a night. I assumed this would be temporary while I was waiting to see what my next career move might be. My first marriage lasted seven years. A few years later I remarried, and my second marriage lasted four years. We adopted my third child, Kelly, who has the most tender loving touch that expresses her giving heart.

I continued delivering papers, enjoying the solitude of being out at night. But over time folding and throwing a thousand news-papers a night took its toll on my body, and my arms, shoulders, and back began to ache. So, at the age of 40, in 1984, I made an appointment for a session of Rolfing, a deep-tissue manipulation that releases and realigns the body and reduces tension, and I loved it! Walking home that day, I experienced my body as if for the first time, and I thought, *I live in a body!* It sounds naive, but when you've spent your whole life shut down, deep-tissue bodywork can be life changing. A few years earlier after reading Carlos Castaneda's book *Journey to Ixtlan: The Lessons of Don Juan,* I remembered the shaman Don Juan telling Carlos something like, "The body never lies," and I was struck by that statement, although I didn't exactly understand it. What I did know was that I needed something in my life that didn't lie to me. Life with my parents had been all lies.

My Rolfer, Nell Luce, and I became friends, then lovers, and not long after we married. And we're still married, nearly 40 years later. Early in our relationship, Nell pointed out something I'd done, and her feedback—amplified and distorted by my defenses—felt life-threatening. I was ready to pounce. As she describes it, I curled my upper lip, I bared my teeth, and with the hot, fierce breath of a rabid dog, I roared back, my contorted face ready to chew her head off. In my first marriage, that kind of rage escalated into long battles about who was right. In my second marriage, the anger created a distance we couldn't bridge. Nell showed me a third way. She ran across the room, put her face right up against mine, and said, "You don't get to talk to me that way!"

Finally, someone was there to help me stop the behaviors that always left me sad and lonely, and a wave of relief washed over my body. Today she's so attuned to these habits that she notices the slightest increase in my volume or a nearly imperceptible curling of my upper lip. And with her support, I've been able to change the physical and emotional patterns I adopted as a child; and I have developed enough sense of safety to be permeable and able to change. It's been a long road, still in process, but I'm now usually able to stay present with whatever I discover within.

After our first Rolfing session, I felt such a relief of tension that I *knew* I had to follow the path of the body, and I became passionate about learning everything I could. I completed the series of ten Rolfing sessions and traveled with Nell to a conference where I met other Rolfers, all embodied in a way that I wasn't. Simply being around them, I could feel my body becoming more aligned. So I told Nell I wanted to be a movement teacher. I was interested in how bodies move and what story those movements might tell us about a person's history and the possibilities of transformation.

I stopped delivering papers to study Rolfing, but the Rolf Institute had just dropped its movement training program. So instead, I spent a year studying the Duggan/French Approach for Somatic Pattern Recognition, also a hands-on bodywork that supports structural, psychological, and emotional alignment. After receiving my certification, I was still too withdrawn and afraid to put my hands on other people's bodies. I could do excellent work, but only on Nell. So I went back to school to study anatomy and physiology; continued teaching myself; and then taught college-level anatomy, physiology, and movement integration at the Desert Institute of the Healing Arts in Tucson.

In 1993, I attended a workshop with Emilie Conrad on Continuum, an approach she created that uses breath, sound, and movement to activate the body's *fluid intelligence* (more about this in Chapter 4, "Continuum and the Fluidity of the Breathable Body"). Within a few minutes of listening to Emilie, I knew Continuum would be my path for life. After the class, I went up to her and said, "I would like to teach this work."

She took a long look at me and said, "You'll have let go of a lot of tension before that will be possible."

I knew she was right, but still, after the workshop I told Nell I'd be teaching with Emilie Conrad within three years. Two years and eleven months later, at another class, Emilie asked if I would like to teach with her. I was beyond thrilled! She recognized the contribution I could make with my knowledge of anatomy and physiology, and thus began an 18-year teaching relationship—creating classes, workshops, and programs—and we became colleagues and the best of friends.

After my first exposure to Continuum, I lightened my teaching load at the Desert Institute and traveled regularly to Los Angeles to study with Emilie and Susan Harper, who was also one of the developers of Continuum; and the two of them helped me open my heart to myself and others. Continuum's profound experiential explorations continue to inform my inner knowing and my teaching. Emilie passed away in 2014, and I still miss her every day.

In 2003, I began a year of studying Buteyko Breathing Education with Jennifer Stark in New Zealand. Buteyko offers breathing exercises as a complementary treatment for respiratory conditions and has helped many thousands of people with asthma, allergies, rhinitis, anxiety, sleep apnea, snoring, and multiple other diseases. And in 2003, I became a Buteyko Breathing educator and later a trainer of Buteyko practitioners. During my time in Tucson, I taught Buteyko Breathing Education to visiting physicians at the University of Arizona's Andrew Weil Center for Integrative Medicine. In the 2010s, after moving to the Pacific Northwest, I continued my study of breathing with masterful teachers Peter Litchfield and Sandra Reamer at the Professional School of Behavioral Health Sciences, and received certification as a breathing behavior analyst.

* * *

In 2012, I was in the Peruvian Amazon lying in a hammock in a small, open-air hut called a *tambo*. The hut was about six by eight feet and had a bed covered by a mosquito net, an open cabinet, a small table and chair, a five-gallon water bottle, and the hammock. I'd been there a week and was beginning to feel comfortable in this remote jungle setting. There were no outside distractions, no sounds from the industrial world; the ecosystem and all the ambient sounds were of nature.

This immersion into pure biological processes stripped away the defenses I usually carry to protect myself from sounds and movements that feel unnatural to me. As each day went by and my defenses peeled away, I began to feel comfortable in my body and safe in the world, at home in the jungle. I'd just come from time along the river watching butterflies, dragonflies, frogs, rocks, plants, and fish dance with each other in perfect harmony. I felt a side of myself I'd never known before—pure joy and a lightness of spirit.

As I lay there, a large red butterfly landed right in front of me on the rope of the hammock. It felt like a "visitation," and I thought, *Wow, I'm going to see this beautiful creature in all its splendor open its wings*. But to my chagrin, it just sat there with its wings closed. I sensed we had not yet developed a relationship that would allow it to show itself in all its beauty and vulnerability, so I settled down and thought, *Okay, let's connect*. I softened my eyes and simply observed, while sending forth heart waves to signal *I'm available. I mean no harm. I'm interested in what we may have in the way of connection.*

Slowly, as I felt myself opening and softening and the intimacy between us beginning to develop, the butterfly's wings began to open and close very gently. I watched and felt, carefully. It took a while; I don't know how long, because time and space were not in my regular reference points. Then, in a moment, the butterfly spread its wings into their full dimensionality of open expression, and in the milliseconds after, my lungs took in the biggest, easiest inhale I've ever experienced.

That moment of expansion contradicted everything I believed about how lungs work. I had thought there was something wrong with me, that my lungs were faulty. Growing up, my lungs always felt constricted. But with that amazing breath, I had a life-changing thought: *There's nothing wrong with my breathing. The* context *of breathing determines how we breathe.* I'd been protecting myself from vulnerability of heart and spirit in inhospitable settings, and now in this safe and natural environment, breath came easily. Asthma was no longer a problem. I was astonished, in love with that moment and the butterfly who delivered this gift then flew away.

A NOTE ABOUT
THE DRAWINGS

---

*Art is more than a passion; it is a tool to heal, transform, and connect.
Riding the wave of breath, a space between arises, a flow state; this is the
place I seek to find in my work. I am deeply honored to work with Robert
Litman, who teaches us to access one of our greatest gifts to health and
consciousness: the breath.*

— JILL ELIZABETH ZIMMERMANN, ILLUSTRATOR

Looking at the illustrations in this book, sense, feel, and imagine how what is being depicted moves in your own body. The images are there so you can look at them and, as you breathe, *feel* what is being shown.

PART I

THE BREATH OF LIFE

Then God, formed a person [Hebrew: adam]
from the dust of the ground
and breathed into his nostrils the breath of life,
so that he became a living being.

— Adapted from Genesis 2:7[1]

CHAPTER ONE

BREATHING *WITH*

All life on Earth depends on Inter-breathing.
All animals breathe in what all plants breathe out;
The trees breathe in what we breathe out.
Our Inter-breathing is the Breath that keeps all Earth alive.

— RABBI ARTHUR WASKOW, AUTHOR AND ACTIVIST

I teach the art and science of breathing. The *art of breathing* is to participate with breath in the movement of life. The *science of breathing* teaches the value of why and how breathing nourishes our organism for better health. Together, they allow us to experience and learn from the breath flowing within us right now.

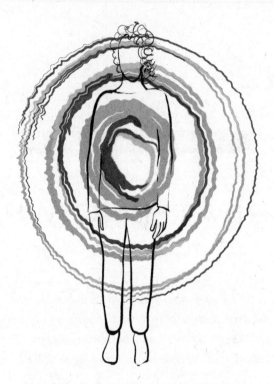

Tides of Breathing: When we inhale and exhale,
subtle waves are traveling throughout the body.

Breathable body means that we breathe with our *whole body*,
not just with our nose or our lungs. Throughout this book, we'll
explore how breathing biomechanics, blood chemistry, and consciousness affect one another, and how they all affect our well-
being. We'll explore ways breathing *habits* and breathing diseases
are shaped over time and their health-related consequences. Most
people are born able to breathe in harmony with the needs of
their cellular life and metabolic activity. But when our emotional
or other primary needs are not met, we adopt strategies for protection, and our breathing changes to guard the tender tissues of our
vulnerable places.

These feelings are "held" in locations throughout the body, and
we consciously or unconsciously expend a lot of energy keeping

them "buried" there. When we begin to notice breath's behavior, we can discover what's going on beneath the surface that needs to be resolved so we can breathe more easily. Practicing this way changes how we breathe and opens us to the joy of being engaged with life.

Over the past three decades, I have moved from teaching *techniques* to encouraging *awareness*. Techniques can alleviate symptoms, and we won't suffer as much. But for change to take hold, we need to allow our bodies and our breathing to *show* us what they need and want. Yoga instructors, bodyworkers, and other health-care practitioners may suggest that we breathe *into* a particular place in our body—to gather more information or to soothe places that hurt. The idea is sound, but I'd like to modify that suggestion: try *breathing with* rather than *into* and see what happens. To me, *breathing with* establishes a collaborative connection between breath and body, and opens a *relationship* with the layers of meaning that are within us.

When breath goes to a painful place, it brings movement and nourishment. Instead of our pain being an *object* to "fix," breath becomes an ally, joining with awareness in a process of discovery. When we breathe *with* a place in our body, we can be present, as with a friend, and receptive to receiving a message of how that place wants to be moved or touched or held.

Please take a moment and breathe *into* a particular place in your body, perhaps someplace that feels tight or hurts. After a few minutes, try breathing *with* the same place and see if you feel more connection. Does "breathing with" change your relationship with that place, and perhaps with your whole body?

When we breathe *into*, we are looking for a specific response, usually release. Breathing *with* opens us to the mystery of awareness—"don't-know mind"—the dance of body and breath. Once we learn to stay present with sensations, our relationship with pain and with our breathable body deepens, encouraging breath's healing powers.

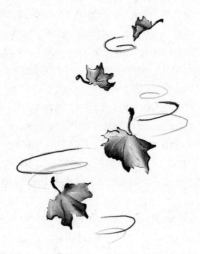

Each breath travels through us in a unique way depending on its flow, texture, speed, and patterning, as well as the physical structure and posture of the body. Like a leaf falling from a tree that spirals to the ground, waves of breath travel through the airways of the body in a spiraling motion. That is the way air moves; the way breath moves; and the way oceans, rivers, and lakes move too. When we hold excess tension, we block this movement, not allowing breath to swirl through the airways of our body, and we limit the nourishment breath can bring.

As I mentioned, most people are born with the ability to breathe freely and naturally, but as the years go by, our breathing can become labored—compromised by disease, fear, disappointment, trauma, and toxins in the air. As a result, defenses express themselves in muscle contraction or laxity, along with shallow or erratic breathing. Over a lifetime of compromises, our breathing capacity becomes less than full.

Consciously *breathing with* our body helps us know when we are operating fluidly and when we're holding, bracing, or shutting down. *Breathing with* isn't a technique or a template; it's an invitation to notice what we need for well-being to return. The inner life of the body is always shifting, according to circumstances. Every breath comes and goes; no two breaths are alike.

Breathing with isn't always comfortable. Over the course of a lifetime, the defenses we build develop into armor by constricting muscles and holding our breath. There are times we cannot continue—touching this landscape may feel too threatening. It's important to rest and recover when we need to and come back when we feel more resourced, safe, and able to tolerate the discomfort buried over so many years, if not generations.

Therapist Matt Licata explains:

> Underneath the narrative of your life, just below the grand storyline, even beneath the colorful emotional landscape, there exists a rich, mysterious world of sensations—a somatically organized field of intelligence and creativity. . . . In any moment, you can infuse your awareness within this field and see very directly that every feeling and emotion—no matter how disturbing or electrifying— is utterly valid, immediately workable, and outrageously creative. It is . . . pure energy, weaved of the magic of dark and of light.
>
> Descending into the body, into this wide open, empty space can seem terrifying, because it is so unknown. You can no longer find many of the familiar reference points from which you come to organize your life. There is no complaining here, no resentment, no "understanding"— not even any "transformation" or "healing" as we have come to think of these terms. Nothing is "unhealed" or in need of transformation. Just raw, naked experience, free from interpretation. . . .
>
> The body is an invitation, an entryway into the freedom, love, and vastness that you are. For it is out of this alive, pregnant crucible of potentiality that flow the qualities of kindness, compassion, attunement, and presence. This is what you are. . . .[1]
>
> Safety first, exploration second, in a dance and dialogue and dialectic that will be unique for each of us. . . . Crafting a safe haven from which to enter into the tender places.[2]

Exploring our inner landscape brings both pleasure and pain, tension and ease. As we learn to explore our breathable body, the stories we tell ourselves about who we are may shift, and we may uncover layers previously hidden. We need patience and an understanding of what we can tolerate and what we can't. Sometimes we need to stop and take a break in order to restore ourselves and self-soothe. I have been practicing this way for decades, and I discovered that what I was most unable to tolerate was not just the darkness and shame but my inner beauty, tenderness, and self-worth. When my mother asked, "What happened to that sweet boy?" I had no idea that I had buried him.

Breathing with the subtle movements of these tender areas, we may slowly reconnect and integrate these vulnerable places back into our wholeness, where they belong. After patiently pursuing the tight spots in my body through breath, the sweet boy is back. I wasn't trying to "fix" anything; I just learned to *breathe with* what is, and I came face-to-face with many shamed and discarded parts of myself. Touching my inner body tenderly with breath, I have regained the treasure of my wholeness, and my life.

Throughout *The Breathable Body*, I will offer short explorations. This is an experiential book, and I hope you will try these explorations, perhaps returning to some of them again and again. Seven explorations are repeated in Appendix G with much more detail. Here are the first two:

EXPLORATION

BREATHING WITH
AWARENESS: "SIMPLY NOTICE"

Notice the air as it enters your body, just below your nostrils, feeling both the air and the movement of your body. *The next breath is right under your nose.*

As you notice the movements of breathing, also *simply notice* that you are aware of being aware. This is your witnessing presence, what Eckhart Tolle describes as your ability "to observe your [own] mind."[3]

Breath, movement, and awareness are in an evolving, mutually beneficial relationship, enhancing your insight into the habits and behaviors of your breathable body, creating the space for you to change habits that no longer benefit your health and well-being.

You can do the same with anything that appears in your awareness: thoughts, images, sensations, feelings, or emotions. Bring a thought or an image to mind while also simply noticing your breathing and that you are aware of both breathing and your thinking. Breathe *with* whatever comes into your awareness.

Breathing is movement. By breathing *with* thoughts, images, sensations, feelings, and emotions, you can see that they too are in movement. Everything comes and goes, including our breathing. Nothing stays. There is only this breath now and what you are thinking, imagining, sensing, or feeling. As breath rests for a moment at the end of the exhale, so do all these other aspects of being human. At the end of each exhale, they dissolve into emptiness. As Eckhart Tolle explains, "Life is now. There was never a time when your life was not now, nor will there ever be."[4]

Everything is moving in and out of existence just like each breath, giving us the opportunity to *simply notice* without having to "do" anything or getting anything "right" or "wrong." All the explorations in this book are meant to be approached with an attitude of "simply noticing" and "breathing with awareness." After you finish each exploration, *simply notice* its effects.[5]

For a longer version of this exploration with additional explanation, see "Breathing *With*" in Appendix G.

EXPLORATION

BEING BREATHED: *Sa~Ha*

You can practice this anytime, anywhere, in any posture that maintains good breathing. (See Chapter 7, "Postures That Support Breath.") There is a longer version of this exploration in Appendix G.

While breathing in, think the sound of the syllable *Sa*; imagine you are saying it, but don't say it aloud. Think one continuous *Sa* for the full length of the inhale. Then, for the length of the exhale, think the syllable *Ha*.

Do you notice anything different from the way you usually breathe while thinking *Sa* and *Ha*? Go back and forth between thinking *Sa~Ha* through the breathing cycle, then not thinking either syllable, to get a comparison. Are you *pulling* air inward when you don't think *Sa*? And when you do think *Sa*, can you feel your *lungs drawing the air into your body*, what I'm calling "being breathed"? When you breathe out with *Ha*, can you feel your lungs releasing the air without you making the effort of pushing the air out? Simply notice.

The purpose of the *Sa~Ha* meditation is to have a quiet and easeful experience of moving air in and out of your body. There are a number of benefits:

- This allows your lungs to draw the air into the body, which may be different from the way you normally breathe.

- It can affect your effort in breathing and increase your capacity for receiving breath by opening the internal spaces more fully.

- Practicing *Sa~Ha* as you inhale and exhale can feel deeply satisfying.

- "Being breathed" by your lungs, rather than by your will or intention, involves 360 degrees. The lungs and torso open and close top to bottom, side to side, and front to back. (See the drawings at the beginning of this chapter.)

- The lungs open from the deepest recesses of their small air sacs and expand outward, breathing *from the inside out*, rather than trying to pull the lungs open.

- This may give you a sense of your lungs breathing you, as they are meant to do, rather than you breathing your lungs.

- With practice, you can learn to make this way of breathing, without constrictions, your default. Eventually, you won't have to think *Sa~Ha*. You'll develop the muscle memory to know how to shift to this way of breathing whenever you sense tension or stress arising and feel a need to soften your breathing and return to a quieter state.

- Breathing while thinking *Sa* and *Ha* can help you access all three openings in the nasal passage, balancing the various functions of the brain. (More about that in Chapter 2, "Your Nose Can Save Your Life," and Chapter 6, "The Anatomy of Breathing.")

- While practicing any of the explorations in this book or anytime in life, you can use *Sa~Ha* or "simply noticing" to bring you more deeply into the present moment.

In 2020, a few weeks after I led a virtual workshop on conscious breathing, I received an e-mail from a senior editor at Hay House who had attended the session and learned the *Sa~Ha* breathing meditation:

> I just finished a 400-mile ultra-endurance, self-supported mountain bike race that took me 89 hours to complete. Dangerously high temperatures were causing mild to severe heatstroke in most racers. The first evening, I couldn't take a deep breath. I'm not sure if it was because I was hunched over on my bike or because of the heat. In any case, the *only* way I could take a deep breath without constriction and a cough was the *Sa~Ha* method. I ended up doing it on and off the bike for the entire race. I'm not sure why, but it worked.

Later, he told me that he practiced *Sa~Ha* while carrying his bicycle up hills that were too steep to ride. He said that while other riders were huffing and puffing, he was having an easy time. In fact, he was one of the few riders who was not exhausted at the end of the day.

I recently recovered from 17 days of COVID-19. *Sa~Ha* meditation kept my lungs open and breathing. Each time I felt breathless and noticed I was trying to breathe from the top of my lungs, I engaged my 360-degree breathing, with my body opening and moving in all directions, top to bottom, side to side, front to back, and all diagonals, using *Sa~Ha*, and was able to bypass the breathlessness.

Some people find it more effective to reverse the order and say, to themselves, "*Ha~Sa*" as they breathe in and out. Please try it both ways, and see what works for you. You can practice these syllables in either order for the *Sa~Ha* explorations throughout the book.

CHAPTER TWO

YOUR NOSE CAN SAVE YOUR LIFE

*Breathe through your mouth as often
as you eat through your nose.*

— JENNIFER STARK, BUTEYKO BREATHING
EDUCATOR AND TRAINER

Jennifer Stark's statement above cannot be overemphasized. Our nose and sinuses are *guardians of the lungs*. They moisten incoming air and can warm it by as much as 40 degrees F (22 degrees C). They filter and clean the air by trapping unwanted particles in tiny hairs called *cilia* and move particulate matter outward in the form of a runny nose or a sneeze or into our digestive tract to be eliminated that way. Nose-breathing also facilitates the production of nitric oxide (NO), an essential bronchodilator that sterilizes the breath in our sinuses on its way to the lungs and acts as an antiviral. And nasal-breathing releases antibodies.

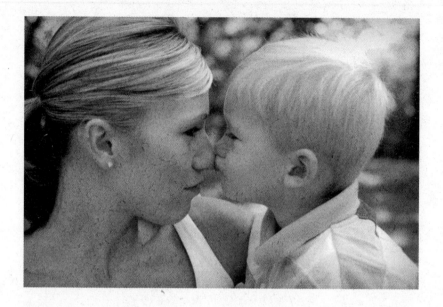

When we breathe through our nose, the air stays in our lungs longer and provides the bloodstream up to 20 percent more oxygen than mouth-breathing does. That may seem counterintuitive, but nasal-breathing *slows* air intake, which is helpful because it requires our lungs to inflate more—taking in more oxygen and supporting lung elasticity. Slower breathing also strengthens our heart and respiratory muscles, and produces a calming effect. Thus, nasal-breathing has a much better chance of supplying needed oxygen to the cells of the body, whereas mouth-breathing is less efficient and can decrease the level of oxygen supplied.[1] In 1931, Otto Warburg won a Nobel Prize in Physiology or Medicine for his discovery of the nature and mode of action of the respiratory enzyme, which demonstrated that only oxygen-starved cells in the body mutate into cancers. Warburg's research has not been replicated or examined in more depth, but his findings hold great potential for future cancer research and treatment.

Nose-breathing can reduce the volume of snoring and sometimes eliminate it, heighten our sense of smell, and support the use of our diaphragm, the primary muscle of breathing. Upon inhalation, the diaphragm contracts and flattens and the chest cavity enlarges. This contraction creates a vacuum, which pulls air into the lungs. Upon exhalation, the diaphragm relaxes and returns to its domelike shape, and air is forced out of the lungs. Smell activates our limbic system, the part of our brain involved in behavioral and emotional responses, so improving this sense with nose-breathing helps us to know what smells safe and what does not. Mouth-breathing, in contrast, can dry the mouth, tongue, gums, and teeth, which can lead to tooth decay and bad breath.

Nasal-breathing also helps attune the electrical activity of the right and left hemispheres of the brain. When we breathe through our *left nostril*, we're tuning the electricity of the brain's *right hemisphere*, which controls the activities of the *left side* of the body. The left side of the body is said to be more receptive, the side that receives information to be processed on the "feeling" level. When we breathe through our *right nostril*, it stimulates the *left hemisphere* of the brain, which helps activate the body's *right side*, which is more the "doing" or active side.

Every 20 to 90 minutes, the body's self-regulating system shifts which nostril is dominant in breathing. This has many implications. For example, sometimes we *think* we should exercise, while in reality we *feel* more like lying around reading a book or taking stock of our emotions. And vice versa: we may want to take time to process our emotions, and our body wants to run around the block. It can be useful to take a moment and feel which nostril is dominant in that moment, as a way of sorting out our impulses.

To find out which nostril is dominant, pinch one closed while breathing in. Then release it, exhale, and breathe in while pinching the opposite nostril. The one that emits a higher pitch is less active in breathing. Another way to tell is to place a mirror or a phone under your nose and breathe out. You will see the vapor on the mirror or phone. The larger amount of vapor comes from the dominant nostril (if there is one—sometimes we breathe out of both nostrils equally).

Strangely, stimulating the armpit appears to affect which nostril is dominant for breathing. I haven't been able to verify this or find an anatomical explanation for it, but it seems to be true. When we lie on our right side, the left nostril is dominant, and vice versa—which is, in part, why we switch sides while we're asleep. Gravity explains a lot of this response. The nostril on top has better drainage and is dominant because of that. Our brain sends signals that it needs a change in stimulus, and we roll over to activate the other nostril for dominant breathing. I heard about a yoga teacher who walked with one crutch, and he would switch which arm he'd use to support the crutch depending on which nostril he wanted to breathe through.

Inside the vestibule (the part of the nose that protrudes from our faces) in each nostril are three bones covered by a mucous membrane that divides the space into three openings: a large space at the bottom, a slightly bigger one in the middle, and a smaller one at the top. These three holes balance brain activity. The lower hole that rides on the opposite side of the roof or your mouth (the "floor" of your nose) is connected to your instinctual reptilian brain. When air moves through this lower hole, the activity of the brain stem is stimulated, bringing bodily functions online. The middle opening is connected to the limbic brain, which is concerned with emotional processing (the heart). And the upper hole connects to the neocortex, responsible for intelligence, spirit, and thought. When we breathe evenly through all three holes, body, mind, and spirit are in balance.

There are times we breathe through one hole more than the others. This can affect our moods and activities. I've observed that people who tend to be uncomfortable feeling emotions and are "in their head" breathe mostly through the top hole. And I've watched athletes about to perform switch to the lower hole to get more energy and power.

Sa~Ha meditation (see the exploration at the end of Chapter 1, "Breathing *With*") allows the lungs time to draw the air of breath through all *three* openings within both nostrils. Breathing slowly while thinking *Sa* and then *Ha* while being mindful of the flow and touch of air makes it possible to feel the air fanning up from the bottom to the middle and top opening. I find that having my brain stem, limbic system, and cognitive mind stimulated by the flow of breath brings me into a sense of continuity and coherence of experience.

Despite all the reasons for nose-breathing, please don't make it a rigid rule and then be disappointed in yourself when, on occasion, you use your mouth to breathe. It takes time to develop a habit, and with effort, at some point you'll find nose-breathing to be as natural, comfortable, and pleasurable as a summer breeze brushing along your cheek. And of course, there are times we naturally use our mouths to breathe—expressing emotions, releasing stress, talking, and perhaps during exercise, although we can learn to exercise while breathing through our nose.

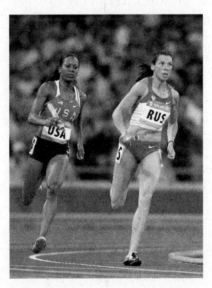

Sanya Richards surges past her Russian rival to help the U.S. win the Olympic gold medal in the 2008 women's 4x400 meters relay, while still breathing through her nose. (Reuters / Alamy Stock Photo)

Structural circumstances, however, can make nose-breathing next to impossible for some people. If that's the case for you, I'd suggest seeing an ear, nose, and throat physician to discuss your options. A deviated septum, collapsed nostrils, or swollen and inflamed turbinates, for example, can make nose-breathing difficult. If you elect to have nasal surgery, I suggest reading about empty nose syndrome, a condition that can result from nasal surgery.[2]

In springtime, when flowers and trees are spreading pollen, some people express allergy symptoms—itchy eyes and runny noses. Pollen irritates our airways, and the outpouring of mucus is the body's way of keeping pollen from entering deep into our organism. Medications that stop mucus production and dry our airways actually increase the disturbance. When our respiratory organs aren't moist, the body won't breathe as much, causing shallow breathing and a sense of being out of breath. In my opinion, it's better to slow down, keep your mouth closed, let your nose run, and just nose-breathe through the river of mucus. Blow your nose gently, as needed, one nostril at a time. You can rinse your nose out with a neti pot or look for a nasal wash bottle at the pharmacy and do copious nose-clearing exercises, including the one at the end of this chapter.

EXPLORATION

MINI-PAUSE

Breathe in and out through your nose. At the end of the exhale, suspend your breathing for three to five seconds; then resume nasal-breathing. This is a Buteyko Breathing Education exercise. Repeat as needed.

Each time you blow your nose, sneeze, cough, yawn, or sigh, you can practice some mini-pauses afterward to reestablish a healthy flow of oxygen and remind the body to breathe from the diaphragm. Doing 15 to 20 minutes of mini-pauses before bed can help reduce nighttime stuffiness. If you are starting to get a cold or while you are not feeling well, try doing 100 mini-pauses within an hour. You can keep track of them by using 100 toothpicks or matches, moving them from one pile to another. I find it easier to take two normal breaths between each mini-pause during the hour. Many have reported, and I've experienced it myself, that doing these has stemmed the onset of the cold. I also used this practice when I had COVID-19 and felt relief. At times when your nose is not too stuffed and is free to breathe, taping your mouth closed at night can help you maintain the benefits of nose-breathing while you're asleep. (More about mouth taping in Chapter 15, "Breathing-Disordered Sleep.")

Nose-breathing and mouth-breathing have different effects on our nervous systems. The parasympathetic branch of our autonomic nervous system has a calming effect ("rest, digest, and settle"), while the sympathetic branch has an activating effect ("fight, flight, or freeze"). The autonomic nervous system is not under our conscious control, although our breathing behavior can affect how it functions. Nose-breathing can bring calming, whereas mouth-breathing can produce activation, anxiety, or even panic.

Imagine a bear coming at you. You take a big gulp of air through your mouth and go into fight-or-flight (or freeze) mode. Your vision narrows so you focus only on the bear. Your heart rate increases to move the blood to your muscles, draining blood from your face and surface skin, and you feel clammy. All nonessential organ activity, like digestion, is turned off, and your immune system goes into overdrive.

Mouth-breathing is part of this lifesaving response and is meant to last only a few moments. Despite the short-term benefits of mouth-breathing in an emergency—it gives us the air we need to act quickly—the air entering our lungs is not receiving the benefits of nose-breathing. When we mouth-breathe more often than we nose-breathe, we trigger these fight-or-flight responses with each breath, and in the long run we increase stress levels, compromising our health.

As a child, I breathed through my mouth, and it affected the formation of my jaw and the alignment of my teeth. Later, when I began studying Buteyko Breathing Education, I made a list of what I was doing when I noticed myself using my mouth to breathe. The list included walking to the mailbox, opening the car door to get out, showering, talking, eating, and doing certain chores like making the bed. Making these activities conscious, I began doing them slowly enough that I could nose-breathe rather than mouth-breathe. Pacing myself helped.

We all mouth-breathe sometimes, but some people breathe through their mouths all the time. There can be many reasons for this, including structural abnormalities like a severely deviated septum or narrow facial features with a high arch in the roof of the mouth. But for most people, mouth-breathing is a learned habit, not a structural necessity. If that's the case for you, try keeping a list of times you notice that you're using your mouth to breathe, noting the activity and your affect or attitude at the time. You can also observe others—the people in your life and public figures in the media—to see whether they mouth-breathe or nose-breathe. Bringing this habit into awareness is a step toward breathing through your nose more. According to a study published in the *European Journal of Social Psychology*, it takes 18 to 254 days to form a new habit and on average 66 days for a new behavior to become automatic.[3]

After you've identified what you're during while you mouth-breathe, try doing the same things while nose-breathing and see if there's a difference. If you're moving through your days quickly and mouth-breathing, slow down. Then pace your overall activity level so you can continue to breathe with your nose. Nose-breathing can save your life.

EXPLORATION

NOSE CLEARING

Having a stuffed nose can cause you to mouth-breathe, which can activate your sympathetic nervous system and disturb your sleep. For those with high blood pressure and heart issues, please limit yourself to six repetitions of this exercise. For everyone else, you practice until you feel a *slight* urge to breathe. Repeat as often as necessary. It's important to read the instructions all the way though before you try it.

- Breathing through your nose, nod your head slowly backward and forward, allowing gravity to do most of the work. You may feel a slight relaxation of your head as it comes to a natural resting position in back, and then in front.

- Try to relax your neck muscles as your head goes forward, and you'll feel a small stretch in the muscles at the back of your neck. Never force the movement.

- Breathe as smoothly, gently, and quietly as possible.

- Slowly coordinate the movement of your head with your breathing: Breathe in, as your head goes back. Breathe out, as your head goes forward.

- Then, keeping your head upright, take a normal breath in and out through your nose.

- At the end of your exhale, pinch your nostrils closed.

- *While suspending your breathing*, tip your head backward and forward three to six times or until you feel a slight urge to breathe. This movement will be faster and more vigorous than before.

- Then release your nostrils and inhale *very gently* through your nose, as if you were trying to receive the subtle scent of a rose.

- Repeat as needed until your nose clears.

If this is uncomfortable for your neck, instead of rocking your head backward and forward, you can stomp your feet while sitting or standing, or walk around the room while practicing. It's the *movement* that creates the change.

It's beneficial to get a feeling for how to do this so that you have the skill when you need it—when your nose is stuffed before bed . . . or anytime.

CHAPTER THREE

THE SENSUOUS NATURE OF BREATHING

Sensation is not considered important, particularly in our Western techno-society, which has moved far away from the river of life and the revelation of the human body. Sensation for most people will circle around pain, sexual arousal, things that feel good and things that don't. . . . [Having an] array of sensation will represent an increased capacity for response.

— EMILIE CONRAD, FOUNDER OF CONTINUUM[1]

While on a walk recently, I turned my attention to the *feeling* of the air around me and noticed that the air's movement was incredibly tender. So I began to breathe with that feeling of tenderness, inviting breath to touch me inside tenderly, and I became *receptive* to the sensuous quality of tenderness. The word *sensuous* comes from the Latin *sensualis*, meaning "endowed with feeling." Breathing is sensual, sensuous, and embodied—endowed with feeling.

Somatically oriented Jungian psychotherapist Sophia Reinders writes:

> I awaken to a fresh, early spring morning and step out into the garden, instantly received by a symphony of fragrances and bird songs. Cool air envelops me, waking up all my senses. I can almost taste its freshness. My gaze wanders to the young birch tree for which I feel a particular affinity. Its pale white branches are softly outlined against the pale blue sky, as they sway in the still air with the gentlest of motions. . . . The first cherry blossoms have opened. I touch my face into them, sensing their soft petals on my skin. Inhaling deeply, I let their light, delicate fragrance fill my lungs. As I listen and sense with my whole body, I feel enveloped in this luminous early morning, vibrating with the aliveness of the first sunlight, the small chirping, clicking, humming sounds of birds and insects, woven together with the fragrances of first blossoms. . . . I feel myself continuous with the living earth. I am filled with gratitude and love.[2]

This is the spirit of the sensuous nature of breathing. Why do we watch animals play, move, hunt, or rest? I believe it's their natural grace—their ease, precision, and flow as they get from here to there. We too are animals with the same capacity. What gets in our way? Self-consciousness? The aches and pains of life's passages? How do we lose our fluid grace, and what can we do to regain the feeling of being at ease and graceful in our bodies?

Animals don't think about or evaluate their performances the way we humans do. They function on instinct, using their senses—smelling, tasting, hearing, touching, and seeing their way through the world, in movement and in rest. They're always in touch with their senses and move in accord with them, which is to say that animals are sensuous, embodied creatures. I think *that* is what we see in their grace—the movement of their sensing, their sensuous nature on display without shame.

We humans can dissociate from our senses when we "live in our heads," concentrating only on thoughts and ideas. There's nothing wrong with thinking, but when thinking disconnects us from sensation, we lose a little of ourselves. Ecopsychologist Michael Cohen observes, "Sense by sense, nature connects with itself in us, through us, and to people and places around us. . . . It validates [the] proposal that *feelings are the truth*, that we don't live in the real world when we ignore what we are feeling."[3]

Breathing is a doorway for us to reenter the natural world of sensations. Breathing in and out, aware of breath's movement and touch, can be a sensuous experience. Inhaling with breath's touch invites our senses to come back online. All our senses are available to guide our grace in movement. What are you seeing, hearing, smelling, tasting, touching, or being touched by right now? What might your senses be telling you about your world?

Sensations are the language of the body. The body records every moment of being alive and stores these experiences in our tissues and deep within our cellular life. Some of what it records becomes conscious, but a lot goes by without our noticing. Nevertheless, it's all recorded and retrievable under the right circumstance, though often in bits and pieces.

After years of holding my sensuous nature at bay, triggered by years of abuse, now when I become aware of my sensuous nature, it settles me and tenderizes the tensions and behaviors that have caused me so much pain. From my experience, the movement toward the sensuous is one of our most profound resources for healing. It's a state of grace. The whole universe participates in our "inter-breathing." We are exchanging energy with the fields that surround us. Breath is breathing us and inviting us to participate.

Respiration is embedded in all of life. The wind that passes over the stones, water, land, and trees and the smells that bring messages of distant lands carry all their stories to the life within us. The currents that began on the beating of the wings of a butterfly also carry the energy of fluttering to remind our hearts of the excitement of life. Each breath cycle carries the universal truth of the currents that make their way into us. The inside environment of our lungs is an extension and undulation of the space outside.

We move along a continuum of breathing patterns from one pole that nourishes us on all levels to another that debilitates and destroys. When we are able to identify where we are on this scale, we can learn to breathe in ways that nourish.

I have spent many years in this exploration of my biology. Continuum explorations are the brilliance that guides me home to my inner life, to the sensuous nature of being animal—the fluids that glide and slide within me, the rich wetland, the sensuous textures that touch me when I'm aware of them in the inner nature of my body. This is our basic nature. Without our senses, we wouldn't be able to navigate life. We wouldn't know what is safe and what isn't. Our brain would not be able to read the signals our sensuous nature is sending it. One of the most disorienting aspects of COVID-19 is the loss of taste and smell.

Our senses bring us pleasure as well as pain. The qualities of eros—love, softness, tenderness, and kindness—hold the frequency of the energy of healing. When I was sick with COVID, I knew intuitively that this was the frequency I needed to have the best chance of transforming the virus's frequency so it would do less damage and give me the best chance to live. This is the rest-and-settle state, being grounded while feeling spacious, kind, loving, and trusting, knowing how to move breath so we can breathe and allow our body to breathe us. In the midst of the huge discomfort, I could feel droplets of pleasure, and this is what kept me from panic and, I believe, from going to the hospital.

My work is to help individuals focus within points of the body that need attention. I teach people how to follow movement and sensations, the relationship between breath and body, and how body and breath interact. With COVID, everything I knew about biology and breathing were tested. Having taught these areas of awareness for decades, suddenly this real-life experience, one that many are having at this time, changed me forever. Breath is life. It's a process of attunement and awareness. Nose-breathing, taking small sips of air when that was all that was available, and being with my sensuous nature were not only sources of pleasure in a time of darkness; they were lifesaving.

EXPLORATION

BREATHING WITH SENSATIONS

Sensations are the language of the body. The sensation *itself* is the message. We *feel* something. Still, it's helpful to have a vocabulary of sensation words so you can describe, to others and yourself, what you feel. See Appendix E for a list of sensation words to get you started. Make up your own too.

Take a baseline, noticing your general state and the quality and rhythm of your breathing. (In the next chapter, "Continuum and the Fluidity of the Breathable Body," I explain in more detail what it means to take a baseline.)

Next, while you are exhaling, feel for any sensations that come into awareness. Continue for a few breaths as you become more comfortable noticing sensations. Then take note of the last sensation you feel as the exhale comes to an end. If you don't notice a sensation, pick any area of your body to focus on.

As you begin the next inhale, keep your attention on that sensation or area while you continue to be aware of the movements of breathing. Imagine that your body is bringing your attention to this sensation because it wants you to understand something about it. As you breathe *with* the sensation, bring a sense of wonder to the area and notice on the next inhalation whether that sensation is the same as or different from when you first felt it. Has there been any movement or a shift in its quality? If the area you're focusing on is painful, is the quality of the pain the same or different? Has there been a change in how your body is moving with breath? Has there been a change in the rhythm of your breathing? Has there been a shift in your sense of being *endowed with feeling*?

Now release this first sensation or area from your awareness and notice the sensation that arrives at the end of the next exhale. *Breathe with* that one for a few breaths and ask yourself the same questions. You can do this for as long as you'd like. When you feel complete, compare how you feel now with how you felt when you began this exploration.

In my mind, each sensation that's calling for my attention wants to be seen and included. These are the places that have become isolated, and they want to receive breath's movement. As they are *breathed with*, they once again become part of the whole. On my best days, awareness itself drops out after a while, and I am "being breathed" with no effort or control on my part. The whole of me becomes a breathable body; there's no longer a distinction between parts and the whole. It's a game of connecting the dots. Each sensation is a dot in my awareness, a location in my body. As breath and awareness connect the dots, a fuller picture of my breathable body comes into view.

I practice "Breathing with Sensations" three times a day for 5 to 20 minutes each time, to restore my naturally slow and quiet breathing rhythm: once in the morning to set the tone for my day, once at midday to decompress, and once in early evening to prepare for a good night's sleep. And I also do it at any time I notice that I need to attend to my inner life to allow what needs to be processed to come to the surface and be integrated, so I can return to my grace-filled sensuous nature.

CHAPTER FOUR

CONTINUUM AND THE FLUIDITY OF THE BREATHABLE BODY

All living processes owe their lineage to the movement of water. Our implicate preexistent memory beginning with the first cell, lies in the mysterious deep, quietly undulating, circulating, nourishing this aquatic being on its mission to planet Earth. God is not elsewhere, but is moving through our cells and in every part of us with its undulating message.

— EMILIE CONRAD, FOUNDER OF CONTINUUM[1]

Continuum was created by Emilie Conrad in the 1960s, with significant contributions from Gary David, Susan Harper, and all the Continuum teachers and students. Each class is a collaboration—an exploration of the inner life of the body using sound, breath, and subtle movements to bring attention to our inner landscape. Continuum is at the foundation of all I am sharing in this book. It's at the foundation of my work as a Buteyko Breathing educator and trainer and as a breathing behavior analyst as well. All the ways I'm inviting you to deepen awareness of your breathable body in the explorations and personal reflections are influenced by my practice of Continuum. Continuum has applications in health care, science, bodywork, meditation, psychotherapy, spiritual practice, business organization, group dynamics, education, dance, artistic creativity, performance, sports, and fitness.

Continuum recognizes that the body is mutable, multifunctional, multidimensional, and without boundaries. What Continuum calls a "body" is *movement*—a dance of cells, molecules, and interpenetrating wave motions. The central teaching of Continuum is that *all* fluids of the body—whether circulating blood, the tides of cerebrospinal fluid, the pump of the lymph system, the net of membranes, or the swirl of viscera and brain—function as a single undulating stream of intelligence. All fluids—whether in the cells, the body, or the planet—are a resonant, intelligent whole, and our lives are sustained by this undulating wisdom.[2]

Inflexibly maintaining stability, even rigidity, can fatigue our tissues and lead to ill health. At a certain point in her explorations with Continuum, Emilie came to realize that watery bodies and fluid psyches have the capacity to heal, nourish, and innovate. She wrote: "Breath is the movement of wind on water—it becomes a beckoning of our origins. As amphibians that developed legs to pursue life on land we return to our watery beginnings."[3]

Emilie's students were reporting changes in how they lived in their bodies, and she wanted to show medical professionals and others that *even when someone is paralyzed*, there is a capacity to feel movement when stimulated through sound; breath; and fluid, wavelike motions. She was not trying to get her paralyzed students to walk again, but she was able to help some of them experience how *movement comes from within* and that feeling their internal moving environment had the potential to shift their identities as nonmoving people.

In one workshop, a woman was wheeled in and had to be lifted out of her chair so she could be on the floor. Later I watched her raise her legs in the air and move them like the arms of an octopus.

Looking closely, I saw *wavelike micro-movements* from deep within flowing through her body, and over the years, I've witnessed movements like this by a number of individuals who had been diagnosed as paralyzed, with no possibility of movement.

Emilie wanted doctors to *see* a paralyzed person move in ways that were unexpected, from the inside out, to validate her principles about Continuum and make a change in the medical community's approach to how to treat paralyzed people and affect the style of rehabilitation. She showed films of these students moving in micro-wave motion, and doctors who worked with paralyzed people simply couldn't understand what they were seeing, so they discounted it. Emilie continued to work with everyone who came to her from far and wide, some moving to Los Angeles for private sessions and to attend her weekly classes.

Emilie saw anyone living in prescribed-movement patterns of body and thought as also paralyzed. Appreciating her perspective, I worked hard trying to notice where I was stuck and how I could bring breath and movement in, and through this practice I've witnessed my own and others' tissues repattern. The inherent wave motion in our bodies can reorganize old patterns, freeing our breathing and opening us to the grace and beauty that is available for us to express ourselves. As I move through old stories and defenses that no longer serve, my compassion for myself and others continues to grow exponentially. Many of Emilie's students have experienced this repatterning, allowing the fluidity coursing through all our bodies to generate movement within, animating our whole being.

I recently watched a seven-minute film clip called "Cheetahs on the Edge—Director's Cut," of a cheetah running at 60 miles an hour in slow motion.[4] Just under its skin, you can see the behavior of the fluid muscles of this incredible being. When it plants its front and rear paws on the earth ever so gently, the fluid muscles are galvanizing, stiffening to support its weight and provide the push-off needed to maintain its speed. When its legs and paws leave the earth, you can see the fluid muscles begin to relax and elongate to their fullest extent. The paws and legs are not drawn back under the body until the undulation of extension is completed. Watching the final extension carefully, you can see the toes waving in the wind, completely relaxed, open, and dissolved from the galvanizing.

The cheetah's head never wavers from its intent of moving forward, with eyes on its prey. The tail is in congruence with the head movement, straight out most of the time, with full elongation through its torso. The cheetah comes into a complete gathering of its tissues, a C curve to gain the power to achieve full extension of its body as it follows through the movement with all four paws off the ground. I watched Caeleb Dressel, seven-time Olympic gold-medal swimmer, reference this clip as a model for how to stay both powerful and relaxed when competing.

Continuum revels in such examples of fluidity and beauty in motion. Continuum is *species-inclusive*. It draws on the evolutionary wisdom that has been passed to us through the bodies of all species. Watching a cheetah run or an octopus undulate can inspire us to explore new ways of moving in our human bodies.

Using Sound, Breath, and Movement to Explore the Dynamics of Breathing

By using sound, breath, and movement to explore the *dynamics of breathing*, we can learn to maximize our breathing potential. *Notice* your breathing as it is now—its rate, depth, and rhythm. Just noticing breath changes it. Take a moment to get an overall impression of how and where your breathing is moving at this moment.

Then sit quietly for a few moments in a way that allows breath to flow easily, not collapsing your chest over your belly. Look directly in front of you with your eyes approximately 10 degrees above the horizon. Try not to look downward, as your head will bend forward.

Be attentive to the speed, rhythm, and depth of your breath again, now that you've been sitting still. Is there a difference?

Perhaps your breath has gotten slower and deeper, and the rhythm has changed. Take another moment to notice the space around your body in all directions. When you do that, do you notice the space inside you as well? Allow your body to settle on what is supporting you—your chair, the floor, a yoga mat, your bed. How might bringing your attention to the movement of breath, your posture, the space around and inside you, and the support beneath you affect the rate, depth, and rhythm of your breathing?

Breath will accommodate changes in posture, behavior, and circumstances. Tracking breathing dynamics can teach us how to be responsive amid the tides of change. Inhaling animates us as our life force returns. Exhaling prepares us for the next inhalation. Breathing can go on unceasingly, repeating this pattern of renewal until our final breath. We arrive into life on an inhale and depart on an exhale. Breathing in and breathing out are repetitions of this cycle. Just as each of us is unique, so is each breath. No two expressions of breath are alike. Whether we are aware of it or not, we never know if there will be another breath. Each is sacred; it is the gift that brings life. When we participate in the dynamic movements of breath and the body, we discover that *breath is a process* and not a fixed pattern.

The explorations throughout this book are not aimed at particular outcomes. They aren't techniques, templates, "shoulds," or even exercises. We're not trying to manipulate breath toward a particular end. We are bringing awareness to the ways our unique breathable body breathes and moves.

The purpose of the explorations is for you to focus attention on and educate yourself about the behaviors of your breathing and their interplay with your physical, mental, emotional, and psychological dimensions. They are all based on Continuum and provide you with a grounded sense awareness. They aren't designed to "fix" anything. They rely on your inner intelligence to reveal, inform, and educate. The simplicity of the practices offered can highlight adaptive patterns from unresolved trauma, dysfunctional breathing, illness, pain, and the general stress of life that may have created constrictions and limitations affecting your breathing, inhibiting its potential to nourish and resulting in physical, emotional, and psychological discomfort.

The explorations allow you to drop beneath the surface noise, stress, and speed of daily life, resting deeply within yourself. As layers of habits and patterns soften, a greater flow of intelligence can guide the body back to its natural state of aliveness. The explorations are sequences of using breath; sound; micro-movements; and nonlinear, spiraling wavelike movements to follow as portals, openings to a deeper awareness of, and connection with, your breathable body, movement, learning, growth, well-being, self-expression, and creativity.

With each breath, our inner life changes. Each time we turn our attention to our inner life, there's something new to discover. We are water beings (almost two-thirds of our bodies is composed of water), and like all rivers, ours is always flowing. Some consider space to be the "final frontier." I believe it's our interiority.

There are two kinds of waves in the ocean: waves that move water and waves that travel through the water. When we're standing on the shore, we see the waves that move water coming toward us. Farther out, even while swimming, we can feel the up-and-down pull of waves moving through the water. In the same way, we have the potential to *feel* these waves of breath traveling through the wet tissues of our body. This way of tracking breath's movement allows us to know ourselves from the inside out.

You are an explorer "diving" into your watery inner world of the breathable body. As you read through the various explorations being offered, you will find many similar instructions. They are there to remind you of how to proceed with a sequence. After a while these will become part of your practice, without the need to read them over and over again.

The explorations may begin to blend together. That's okay. You can mix and match what brings you the best results. At first it is good to stay true to the sequence as you get a feel for the process. Each exploration is a practice in and of itself and is meant to be repeated often to enhance the conscious development of your relationship with your breathable body and your ease with breath.

At the foundation of it all are the specific movements, sounds, and breaths that are uniquely yours—tuning in to your own breathable body and fluid intelligence. In the explorations, I'm simply presenting invitations to help you deepen awareness and presence with your own unique breathable body.

Like all watery landscapes, our inner landscape is fluid. It changes based on prevailing winds, the ebbs and flows of tides, and other predictable and unforeseeable factors. The human landscape is more or less the same for all humans—the arrangement of our organs and how the elements of our system communicate with one another. What makes each of us unique are the physical and emotional hands we've been dealt, how we've responded to them, the nutrients we ingest, and the conditions that surround us. Our inner landscape is a living *process*. With that in mind, please continue to try the short explorations throughout the book and the longer ones in the Appendix.

BASICS OF CONTINUUM

Taking a Baseline

Every exploration in this book begins with a *baseline* inquiry to help you notice what's true for you as we start, and each exploration ends with a comparative inquiry so we can see what has changed in you as a result of the exploration. A baseline is, by definition, "a starting point used for comparisons." In this context, baselines are observations of the details of your breathing and physical and emotional states in the present moment. Comparing beginning baselines with ending states is an interoceptive inquiry (delving into how your body feels inside) to help you understand how you have changed and what you have learned from this practice.

Please take a baseline as you begin each exploration. Here are some questions you might ask to get the lay of your *inner landscape*.

You don't have to answer all of them. It's fine to focus on one or two, or just respond to whatever else you notice.

- What's on my mind now?
- How am I feeling emotionally?
- How am I feeling physically?
- What else is interesting to me in this moment?
- What matters most to me at this moment?

After asking yourself questions like these, turn your attention to the *quality* and *dynamics* of your breathing and how your body is responding to the movement of breath. Then ask yourself:

- What is the speed, pace, depth, and rhythm of my breathing?
- What are the *qualities* of my breathing—for example, the density, texture, and volume?
- Am I using my mouth or my nose as I inhale and exhale?
- What is the sound of my breathing?
- Am I controlling my breathing, or am I allowing breath to rise and fall on its own?
- Where do I feel my body moving in response to my breathing?
- Where does my body touch the surface beneath me, the ground that is supporting me?
- What is my perception of the space around me and within?
- Do I notice recurring habits that may limit my breathing?

Each time you take a baseline and a follow-up inquiry, you increase the knowledge of your experience. You can also take baselines throughout the day by noticing whatever arises in your awareness about your body, mind, and spirit/breath. What do you notice now that may be new? Changes in your breathing, thoughts, or behavior since your last baseline? Taking note (simply noticing breath by breath) can transform your world and your life.

Sensation

Sensation is the language of the body. It is the basis for every exploration baseline: What do you feel? What do you sense? When you're aware of a sensation, you are feeling. You don't have to diagnose what you feel. Simply notice. Just feel it. The explorations are designed to stimulate sensations and your awareness of them. Learning the language of the body allows you to speak clearly about your experience and to know what your body is trying to tell you.

Sequences, Open Attention, and Layering

After you take a baseline, follow the exploration's instructions, which will be a series of steps. Going through an exploration once is called a *sequence*. At the end of the first sequence or at any time you feel like investigating the impact an exploration is having on you, practice *open attention*, which means to invite into consciousness whatever has been stimulated by breath, sound, or movement to help it be integrated. Open attention is also the time to feel for and follow any impulses for movement that may be different from the way you usually move. This is not a time for judgment, just the elegant simplicity of discovering whatever arises in your awareness. Notice whatever old patterns or new perspectives you are experiencing. It's a time to be informed and affected.

When you feel you've spent enough time in open attention, you can repeat the sequence. This is called *layering*, and it too is followed by open attention. During the second layering (which is the first sequence repeated, although invariably new responses will arise and outcomes will be different), your attention is likely to be more focused. If you decide to do a third layering, keep the instructions in mind, but at this point follow your impulses and be mindful of patterned behaviors or predetermined ideas.

During the first sequence, follow the instructions as you become acquainted with your inner realms and familiarize yourself with them. In the second and third layerings, particular aspects of the sequence or areas of the body may draw your attention, and you can spend more time there. After the third round, allow a longer period for open attention, and you may discover that you're feeling a deeper intimacy with yourself. Simply notice what is present, and then after a pause, take another baseline, compare it to the baseline you took at the very beginning, and note what has changed and what you've learned.

If you only have time for one layer, comparative observing will come after that. If you do two sequences, it's at the end of the second one. If you do three, it comes at the end of the entire exploration. Doing this can help to modify habits and encourages a gentler, more nourishing flow of breath and body.

Scaffolding

Another term used in Continuum—*scaffolding*—means "noticing how structures within the body rest on each other and move in relationship with the whole body." For instance, the heart rests on the diaphragm, and the organs of elimination settle into the pelvis. When you raise your arm and move it like a tentacle, you may feel its reverberating movement through your torso and perhaps down your legs. Building a scaffold means becoming aware of the ways these internal parts are resting, settling, and connecting with one another, building a unified and coherently responsive structure from head to toe. Building an inner scaffold can transform you from feeling fragmented to feeling unified and coherent.

Sound

Sounds are audible breath. Air passing through our vocal cords produces sounds. Hans Jenny, a physician, studied the acoustic effect of sound waves on various materials and observed that different frequencies of sound create different patterns in matter. He called this new science *cymatics*. Sound moves molecules and organic materials, including the tissues of our body, changing densities to create more space and permeability. When we hear sounds from the outside or sounds that we ourselves make, we can feel the vibrations that are moving in our bodies, and they affect us.

Making a sound can be difficult for some people. You may have been mocked or scolded about your voice, and now you're shy about expressing yourself, scared of what others might think. When I was in sixth grade, I tried out for glee club, and I was so frightened that my voice croaked. The teacher rejected me, and I considered myself unworthy of ever singing again. It took time and effort for me to feel comfortable enough with others in a Continuum class to produce sounds like the ones I'm suggesting to you. Be patient and go as slowly as you need to. Begin in a space where you're alone, where no one else can hear you. Once you feel safe enough, try to access the range of vocalization your body can make. Sounds are like flashlights illuminating and bringing awareness to internal aspects of the body. When you use sound in the sequence, take the time to notice the vibrations (sensations) they produce and how the sound may be affecting your experience.

For most explorations that use sound, I suggest humming or pronouncing a vowel, usually a long *O* or a long *E*. Vary the pace and allow your awareness to ride the tide of the sound. You can direct the sound to particular areas of your body, send it on specific trajectories, or let it travel wherever it may.

As Hans Jenny discovered, when you create sound, vibrations literally enter your tissues, shifting molecular arrangements, *helping your body become more breathable*, and over time the range of motion and the capacity to accommodate breath increase. No two sounds are identical. Each audible breath leads to a new experience within you. Go slowly and find sounds that please you. As your body softens and becomes more breathable, the more sustained your sound will be.

The patterns of our breathing and the sound of the breath express the way we feel. When someone is crying or laughing, the sounds of grief or joy are carried on their breath. We can even hear or feel the suppression of emotional expression. There may be a tightness in the voice or a halting pattern. We can feel it in our body as we listen. Breath is meant to be silent. Whether it is silent or carries a sound, it is relaying a message about our internal state.

Touch

All the explorations in this book activate our interior sense of being touched, including the touch of the movement of breathing. In addition, some of the explorations invite us to touch our body with our hands, such as the belly exploration or discerning whether our inhale inflates our chest or our abdomen first. Self-touch helps us gain more awareness in the areas we are exploring.

When you are about to touch your body, ask yourself if it's okay. Go slowly and honor your ease and your discomfort with self-touch. Approach your body with respect and listen to yourself if touching at that moment does not feel within your "window of tolerance," an expression introduced to me by writer and somatic therapist David Treleaven regarding trauma-sensitive mindfulness. When you return to these practices over time, touch might feel easier. Touch lightly, but with enough pressure to feel the movement beneath your hands. Pushing too hard, though, may dampen sensing and movement.

Wave Motion

Life probably began in the ocean at least 3.5 billion years ago. Constituents of these life-forms, all floating separately in the sea, over time became multicellular organisms. Like people at a concert today, they came into proximity with one another, and the undulating wave movements of the water mixed and stirred them all. Photosynthesis began more than 2.5 billion years ago—the Great Oxidation Event—but it took hundreds of millions more years for enough oxygen to build up in the atmosphere and the oceans to support complex life. Below the surface of our awareness, these primordial waves continue within us (and within every living being), moving materials in and out of our cells—enabling life and facilitating growth. The waves generated by our breathing move these inner waves, as Emilie would say, "like wind over water." Breath is the initiatory wave.

When a section of a river stops flowing, the water stagnates, eventually drying up. When there's stagnation in the body, those areas become painful and stiff. In modern culture, when we develop musculoskeletal problems, many health practitioners prescribe linear movements to restore function through bending, flexing, and extending. These can be extremely useful, but in my experience, tuning in to the undulating, spiraling, curving, and arcing interior waves that already exist inside us can be the beginning of a deeper healing.

Micro-Movements

Micro-movements are nearly imperceptible movements. After bringing sound, touch, or breath to an area, you may notice tiny movements there. The micro-movements we value in Continuum practice are the ones that are coherent, travel in wavelike motions, and bring awareness to an area of interest, helping us experience how the smallest movements can engage our fluid network. A micro-movement that can also be initiated in one location may travel to another place in the body, near or far, or through your whole body all at once.

Be curious about how small a movement you can make and still feel it traveling. Feel the tiniest twitch of your nose or cheek. This is the body's capacity for communication and healing within. Micro-movements are most effective when you feel still and quiet. If you're distracted or activated, they'll be harder to notice. When a micro-movement travels through a pathway, *the wave of breath follows*. When you notice this, your breathable body will soften and become more responsive to breath's movement.

EXPLORATION

INCREASING BREATHING CAPACITY WITH SOUND

After taking a baseline, make a "hum" sound on the exhale. Practice until you find a sound that soothes and that you consider pleasing.

Notice how the sound's vibrations travel in your body. Can you feel them? Where in your body do you notice these vibrations? They will follow their own path and, in so doing, draw your attention to particular locations. Focus on one of these locations as you inhale and exhale. Is this place *moving* in response to breath? Breathe *with* that location for two or three breaths. This is similar to the exploration with sensations, but this time you are creating the sensations with your humming.

After each audible breath, take two or three silent breaths until you have the breath to make another sound. While breathing silently, notice if there are any differences from breathing with sound. Then practice open attention.

After that, do another "hum" on an exhale, and repeat this inquiry at least six more rounds or for as long as it feels comfortable and not effortful.

As breath begins to move where the vibrations land, the quality or tone of each sound may be different from the time before, as the resonant chamber of your body is growing more dynamic. The sound you are making may change pitch, volume, and length. Play with the quality of the sound by making it bigger or lengthening or shortening it. Use the sounds E and O for variety. For more awareness, you can place your hands where you feel the vibrations moving.

Feel if the quality of your breathing has changed. Does playing with sound have an effect on your breathing? Is your body more open and responsive as you breathe in and out? Has the effort of breathing changed? How is your breathing capacity? Do you have more room to breathe? How is the ease of flow?

During the day when you need some time to connect to yourself, you can repeat this, or add it to any other explorations to increase awareness.

There is a more extensive version of this exploration, "Sound Practice," in Appendix G.

EXPLORATION

WAVE MOTION

Water carries within it the intelligence of the sensuous. Its sensuous texture is one of its gifts, and the animal sensing part of us knows this. This is an exploration of wave motion—working with water's *intelligence* and its undulating wave forms. As we become aware that these waves are (literally) always moving within our bodies, including waves of breath, the waves themselves will guide us toward an impulse to undulate, awakening new options for grace in movement.

For this exploration, we'll use the long vowels *E* and *O* and/or a humming sound. Use one sound for all three sequences, or vary the sound layer by layer or within one layer. For example, in layer two you may start with a humming sound for two breath cycles, then switch to a long *E* for two breath cycles, then a long *O* for the last two rounds of sound and breath. Using different sounds, you'll discover what you feel most comfortable with and which are most effective in sensing different areas of your body. As with all explorations, there is no predetermined result. Everyone is different, and each time will be different from the times before.

First Layer: Awareness–Breath

Begin with a baseline. You will be observing how using sound, breath, and wave motion changes your experience of yourself, your breathing, and the movement of your body.

Pick a place in your body you feel drawn to explore, a place accessible to both hands. *Breathe with* that place for a round of six or more breathing cycles. Then rest in open attention and notice what comes into your awareness: thoughts, images, sensations, or any meaning you are making of your experience.

Second Layer: Breath–Sound–Touch

Begin the same way as layer one. Stay with the same location in your body.

Place your hands there while making a "hum" sound, the sound of *O*, or the sound of *E*. Repeat for six rounds of sounding and touching, and each time you finish making the sound, *breathe with* where you feel the vibration under your hands for the next two or three breaths before beginning another round of sound and touch.

At the end of six rounds of touch, sound, and breath, open your attention without focus, just being curious about what comes into your awareness. Don't look for anything specific and you may be surprised what shows up.

Third Layer: Breath–Sound–Touch and Wave Motion

Make sound with the tissues of the same location a few times until you feel a vibration under your hands with either a "hum" or an *O* or an *E* sound. After each sounding and breath, focus on the *shape* of the area under your hands, and breathe with that shape, as though you were filling it with breath. Feel the dimensions of the shape, especially the edges, from left to right, back to front, then from top to bottom—all dimensions. As you breathe with the shape, continue to sense how breath fills and moves the dimensions. Do a few rounds of sounding with both hands on your body, and breathe with the sensations and shape of the area. When you get a sense of the shape, imagine it filled with water (which, actually, it is, since the tissue under your hand is mostly water), and with a small amount of pressure from your hands, push the water back and forth in a way that moves it from side to side, creating a wavelike movement.

Move the water to one edge, and then wait until you sense/feel that it has arrived at the opposite edge. Then send the water back to the first side, waiting until you sense/feel it has arrived there. Keep sending waves back and forth under your hands, as if you are sloshing water inside a bowl. The water goes to one side and back to the other.

Then feel whether you can touch all the edges from side to side, front to back, diagonally, and top to bottom, filling the space with micro-wave motions. This wave is traveling through the water. After a few moments of pushing the fluid under your hands back and forth and around, remove your hands and feel if you can create the same micro-wave movement without using them, just by undulating your body. Play with that idea and movement for a few moments. You are learning how to use wave motion to have more awareness of your body, increasing the capacity and fluidity of the movements of your breath and body.

Rest in open attention. Don't focus on anything; simply notice what arrives into consciousness. This is information to harvest.

After the last layer, notice how you are feeling and compare it with the baseline you took when you started. Feel the capacity of your breathing—its ease or non-ease. How is your body breathing? How are you perceiving yourself and your breath? What have you learned about attending to yourself and helping your body open and receive the movement of breath? Notice if this deepens your experience that no two breaths are exactly alike and if you have a sense awareness that *everything* comes and goes along with each breath.

It can be useful to keep a journal of these explorations. Sometimes writing down our discoveries opens us to further insights.

CHAPTER FIVE

THE WORLD
IS ON FIRE

The air we breathe is essential to human life, yet we often take it for granted. In Canada alone, air pollution is responsible for causing thousands of deaths, millions of cases of illness, billions of dollars in health care expenses, and tens of billions of dollars in lost productivity every year.

— DAVID SUZUKI, SCIENCE BROADCASTER
AND ENVIRONMENTAL ACTIVIST

At the November 2022 United Nations Climate Change Conference (COP27), Egyptian artist Bahia Shehab invited visitors into two unlabeled rooms. One had a light, domed interior set at a comfortable temperature in the low to mid-70s Fahrenheit, surrounded by nature sounds and scents of "freshness, orange blossoms." The other was a dark, claustrophobic space set around 95 degrees Fahrenheit, reeking of decomposing fruit and hospital rooms. She called these "scenarios of eternity," representing two possible outcomes for humanity. She intended to give visitors a visceral experience of the choices we face about global warming, and called the exhibit "Heaven and Hell in the Anthropocene."[1]

According to the World Health Organization, 99 percent of the world's population now lives in places where air pollution exceeds safe limits, and the UN has identified air pollution as the largest environmental risk to global public health.[2] As of May 2022, COVID-19 had been responsible for 15 million "excess deaths,"[3] and a Harvard study found that in places with higher air pollution, there was an 11 percent increase in mortality for every microgram-per-cubic-meter increase in air pollution.[4] This period of time is called by some the Pyrocene Age.[5] Our planet is burning, and the air we share is becoming unbreathable.

On a recent car trip from Seattle to San Francisco, my wife and I were blinded by smoke from a series of wildfires along Interstate 5. There was so much smoke we could barely make out the iconic shape of Mount Shasta. When we got out of the car, our eyes were burning and we both choked, which triggered in me the dread that asthma could kick in at any moment. We put on our masks, not for COVID but to keep the smoke out of our lungs.

We live on Vashon, a small island in the Puget Sound, near Seattle. Four years earlier, in the summer of 2018, wildfires throughout the Pacific Northwest blew in so much smoke that we couldn't see 10 feet in front of us. Looking up, the sun was bright red. I knew the fires weren't on our island, yet I felt a kind of primal fear. During two weeks of heavy smoke, Nell and I limited grilling, frying, and baking, which can bring indoor air quality to hazardous levels in a matter of minutes. Opening windows was not an option, so we used a microwave, steamed some foods, and ate foods that didn't need to be cooked. We stayed quiet, sitting in comfortable positions so our lungs were not compressed by our bellies. With less physical stress, we automatically breathed less.

In early 2020, over 14 million acres of land were burning in Australia. Over a billion animals likely perished there, with temperatures reaching 120 degrees F in some areas. In the western U.S., the average wildfire season is now 78 days longer than it was in 1970 and burns more than twice as much acreage, almost certainly due to climate change. There are countless other examples in recent years of extreme forest fires—in the Amazon, throughout

Europe, and even in the Arctic. A 2021 study indicated that wildfire smoke affects respiratory health more than fine particles from other sources.[6] A study published in *The Lancet* in May 2022 found that people who lived within about 30 miles of a wildfire in the last decade were about 5 percent more likely to develop lung cancer and 10 percent more likely to develop brain tumors than those living farther away.[7]

And it's not just wildfires. According to the National Parks Conservation Association, the air quality in 85 percent of U.S. national parks is "unhealthy."[8] Shanghai, Beijing, Los Angeles, Delhi, and many other cities have unhealthy air almost daily. In Delhi, people insert filters into their nostrils and wear masks. A study co-authored by the U.S. National Institutes of Health showed that in Shanghai, college students who were given air purifiers for their rooms for 48 hours demonstrated clear cardiopulmonary benefits. Those who didn't developed inflammatory damage to their lungs, heart, and blood vessels. What's being measured is nitrogen oxide, sulfur oxide, carbon dioxide, carbon monoxide, and ozone. Ongoing exposure to unhealthy air kills one in six people worldwide.[9]

As I complete the writing of this book in 2022, respiratory diseases like Acute Respiratory Disease Syndrome (ARDS) and Respiratory Syncytial Virus (RSV) are rampant, due in significant part to humans and other life-forms breathing air that debilitates our immune systems and makes us more vulnerable to the many viruses traveling in the air worldwide.

The symbol $PM_{2.5}$ ("particulate matter 2.5") refers to tiny particles or droplets in the air that are two and a half microns in width or less. There are about 25,000 microns in an inch. The largest of these particles are about 30 times narrower than the width of a human hair. $PM_{2.5}$ causes inflammation, which gives rise to acute and chronic respiratory disorders, lung cancer, heart attacks, strokes, and an increased risk of diabetes. The combined effects of ambient air pollution and household air pollution is associated with seven million premature deaths annually.[10] World Health Organization data shows that almost all of the global population (99 percent) breathes air that exceeds WHO guideline limits and contains high levels of pollutants, with low- and middle-income countries suffering from the highest exposures.[11] London researcher Sefi Roth found that the variation in average results were staggeringly different. The most polluted days correlated with the worst test scores. On days where the air quality was cleanest, students performed better.[12]

Air pollution is likely a causative factor in many inflammatory diseases that are being labeled idiopathic, or of unknown origin. When the air is unhealthy or smells bad, a *healthy response* is for our lungs to limit their breathing capacity, which results in us learning to become shallow- or mouth-breathers. But when the air is toxic over time, stressed breathing weakens our immune system, heart, and lungs, and we may become breathless, expressing symptoms such as asthma, anxiety, sleep disturbances, generalized aches and pains, high blood pressure, heart abnormalities, and mental fatigue. There is a rise in childhood and adult-onset asthma. The elderly, the poor, the houseless, people of color, and other marginalized populations are the most likely to have compromised health. According to Rupa Marya and Raj Patel, authors of *Inflamed*, "Inflammation is a biological, social, economic, and ecological pathway, all of which intersect, and whose contours were made by the modern world."[13]

The constituents that make up our atmosphere are changing. What we breathed in when our species' lungs developed, or even when I was growing up in the mid-20th century, was much different from the air today. Coal miners brought canaries into the mines to tell them when the air was too dangerous to breathe. If a canary died, they knew it was time to leave the mine. More people are suffering from respiratory distress today than at any other time in history, approximately 20 percent of the population, and the largest portion of these are children, the elderly, and people diagnosed with sensitive airways. The World Health Organization says that pollution kills more than 1.7 million children under the age of five per year.[14] They are the canaries in our coal mines, letting us know that the air we're breathing is becoming hazardous to our health. Knowing how to breathe effectively and how to create a clean, safe environment at home can help to a large extent, but remedial responses don't hold a candle to coming together as a world community to re-create an atmosphere of clean air.

Nearly every news story and thoughtful conversation about global climate change focuses on the impacts of increased carbon in the atmosphere—ice caps melting; sea levels rising; out-of-control weather systems leading to fires and floods, heat waves and blizzards. But we hear less about how the changing atmosphere is *already* affecting breathing and health.

Polluted air is everywhere, and our bodies, collectively, are already feeling the effects. For political leaders and whole populations to get the message that *change is needed now,* the effects of breathing toxic air must be recognized as both extremely dangerous and a result of climate change. We need to work with health-care professionals to address our individual breathing disorders, but to address atmospheric health, we need activism, finding a way to enact worldwide agreements to address these existential and public health issues. Deeply knowing and feeling—in our bones and in our lungs—the effects of hazardous air quality can bring everyone into the vast global grassroots movement needed to reverse climate change and clean up the air we share.

There are ways to mitigate the effects of poor air quality, although they are far less effective than leaving fossil fuels in the ground. When the air turned bad on Vashon in the summer of 2018, I made sure I used only my nose for breathing. The human nose traps particulate matter greater than .5 microns ($PM_{.5}$), combining them with mucus for elimination. I rinsed the inside of my nose with water after coming in from outside. This provided a little help, but unfortunately, smoke and the gases from smoke (including carbon monoxide) are less than .5 microns and go right into the lungs, heart, blood vessels, and other organs. So I needed more protection.

I purchased an indoor air-quality monitor to track the air throughout our home and a purifier for each room to filter the smoke, gases, and particulate matter smaller than $PM_{2.5}$, adding a high-efficiency particulate air (HEPA) filter with an activated-charcoal filter to eliminate odors, smoke, and gases smaller than .5 microns. Do-it-yourself air purifiers can be made by combining a fan with a household furnace filter.[15] I bought masks rated by the National Institute for Occupational Safety and Health (NIOSH) at N99, which means they can filter up to 99 percent of $PM_{2.5}$ from the air, each with a release valve to remove excess heat and moisture while exhaling and allowing additional activated charcoal to be inserted. All these precautions can be put into place starting at around $50. The cost of air monitors has also come down, and some air purifiers have air monitors built in.

To ensure that my home was smoke ready, I created what the EPA calls a "clean room," one that is smoke-, gas-, and particulate-matter-free. The air monitor gave me the information to ensure that each room was clean. I checked for leaks at the windows and closed all vents open to outside air. And I placed a towel at the bottom of the doors to the outside when I was indoors and at the bottom of the bedroom door on the outside when I went out.

Breathing well, especially while sleeping, is the basic step in giving the body a chance to allow the immune system to cope. A client recently told me, "When I slow down my breathing and reduce the volume of air, I breathe from a deeper place within, and I feel like I'm breathing through a straw."

This is a keen observation on two counts. First, she could sense that when she initiated her breathing from a deep layer rather than superficially trying to grab air in desperation from the belief of needing more, her breathing slowed down, became quieter, and most importantly, passed through her airway without effort.

Breathing from a deep place within allows the diaphragm to move downward, pulling the lungs open to draw in the air and the chest to expand to further support that process. Then, during the exhale, allow these structures to relax and release the air without effort. *Sa~Ha* breathing meditation teaches and reminds the body to use the primary respiratory muscles for breathing, rather than using neck, upper back, and facial muscles to pull air into the body. The nose, as guardian of the lungs, regulates the flow of air, and this process of moving air quietly and slowly engenders peacefulness, setting the tone for a day worth living. With somatic awareness, we become clear about our need for clean, breathable air.

There are ways to minimize the damage being done to our lungs in the short run with filters, monitors, and conscious breathing. But equally, and probably far more important, is the renewal of our appreciation of the sacredness of breath so we will do whatever we can to contribute to the massive environmental and lifestyle shifts needed now. *Feeling* the atmospheric changes already underway may be key to dismantling denial. I hope everyone will join in the immense effort needed to enact a very Green New Deal to create again, over time, a breathable biosphere.

There are precedents for nations coming together to improve the quality of the air. The UN Montreal Protocol, finalized in 1987 and ratified by every country in the world, has phased out 98 percent of the world's ozone-depleting substances, with an estimated two million people saved from skin cancer every year. By 2019, just 12 years after the protocol's ratification, the ozone hole was the smallest since its discovery, and it's expected it will return to pre-1980s levels by the middle of the 21st century.[16]

Another success, although short-lived, took place right after the arrival of COVID-19, when halts in manufacturing; reductions in air, cruise-ship, and car travel; and other emissions stoppages freed the air of pollutants more than any time in decades. In a matter of weeks, the air and sea were cleaner and horizons more visible than they'd been in decades, and we got a glimpse of what it would be like to have clean air. In August 2022, President Biden signed a bill investing $369 billion in clean energy, including a 40 percent reduction in carbon emissions by 2030. This is the biggest piece of climate legislation in American history (so far).

Transforming our world and ourselves one breath at a time begins by realizing the depth of our interconnection with each other and our planet. And it all starts with the sacred act of breathing—feeling the blessing of each inhalation and exhalation.

EXPLORATION

IMAGINE

Take a moment to sit quietly and breathe with your imaginings of a world where everyone has:

- Enough clean and healthy food to eat

- Fresh, clean, crisp water

- Fresh air that has no odor other than the smells of nature

- Shelter from the elements, secure in its structure offering a safe harbor of protection

- Exposure to sounds that are only biological; industrial sounds are nonexistent

- The sight of only friendly faces and clear vistas

- Nothing out of place in the life-and-death cycle of all things

Place yourself there, wherever that might be for you. A beach, a jungle, the mountains, a valley, a desert. Fill in as much detail as you can, from memory or imagination. Picture it peopled with those you love and who love you. You are free to be your most essential self. No veils are needed to protect you.

Each time you notice that you feel pleased by what you have created with your imagination and your senses, notice how you are breathing. How it might have changed from the way you normally notice your breathing. How your body and breath play together to create the space and flow to nourish this state that you have dropped into.

Then go on creating this perfect haven. Discover yourself within the harmony of your creation. When you have made this home for yourself and feel complete, rest back and breathe, drift and dream.

PART II

FUNDAMENTALS OF BREATHING

Outside it's air

Until you breathe in, inhale

And then inside, air becomes breath

— Diana Farid, *When You Breathe*

CHAPTER SIX

THE ANATOMY
OF BREATHING

The human body is simply the most beautiful complexity.

— ATTRIBUTED TO DANIELA ISMERIO, M.D.

While I was training in the Duggan/French Approach for Somatic Pattern Recognition, the teachers suggested that I study anatomy. Since I've always loved biology, studying anatomy seemed like a great next step. So, during the winter break in my training, I traveled to Chicago and studied for 10 days with Jon Zahourek in his program of Anatomy in Clay. Jon had developed anatomically correct 12-inch skeletons that we could work with at our tables. Over the course of a week and a half, each of us built all 600-plus muscles of the human body on our mini-skeleton. Jon's motto was: "The mind cannot forget what the hands have learned."

Imagine building the entire muscular body from the deepest to the most superficial muscles and not have it looking like the Hulk. You have to be precise as to the size and dimensions of *each* muscle. If you make one too large, the next layer of muscle will also be out of proportion. Jon's motto proved true for me. I have never forgotten what I learned in that class, and it laid the foundation for all my future anatomy study.[1]

When I finished my training and became certified in the Duggan/French Approach, the owner of the massage school in Tucson where I had been teaching movement integration suggested I teach college-level anatomy to her massage-therapy practitioners. So I taught for three hours twice a week, and had to study about 30 hours a week to be able to do so. Nell would come home and find me surrounded by a dozen or more anatomy books—I was learning from different authors' perspectives. I even read the U.K. edition of *Gray's Anatomy*, over 1,200 pages, from cover to cover. I was dedicated and fascinated.

At first I thought I had to memorize every detail and hold it all in my mind. At the time, I was an avid reader of detective novels. Then one day I realized I simply couldn't memorize that much detail; it's too complex and too layered. So I began to treat the study of anatomy as a detective might. I'd study one layer, or one perspective, until I *understood* how each structure fits into the whole. After that, I would *feel* each layer and how it moves in my body in concert with the others. By the time I went to teach the next class, I was sharing from experiences *in my body*, which made the teachings relevant for the students and for the clients they were massaging.

As part of the class, I took the students to the dissection laboratory at the University of Arizona, and the lab professor guided us through dissections. After the first dissection, my mind was turning quickly like cogs on a wheel. Everything I had studied and learned from the books was being reorganized into three-dimensional perspective. Anatomy was never the same for me after that. It was real, reinforcing what I'd learned in Jon Zahourek's Anatomy in Clay class, this time including my own somatic experiences as well. The pieces began to fall together, and I could see it all as a living process of connections, movement, and growth.

After completing *The Breathable Body* manuscript, while awaiting the publisher's response, I tested positive for COVID-19, as I've mentioned before. Nell did too. We had both received two doses of the Moderna vaccine and one booster, although the booster had been almost a year earlier. What a ride! Without knowing what I know about anatomy and the physiology of breathing, I don't know what I would have done to stay sane and out of the hospital. It hit us both pretty hard, and I am changed, probably forever, by this force of nature.

COVID-19 comes not only with respiratory challenges but with the stories about so many people dying or having long COVID, being debilitated for months, if not years. Along with being quite sick, we were both really scared. I'm asthmatic, as I've also mentioned, and the first way the virus caused me difficulty was a tightening in my chest. As I had for so many years, I was once again coughing into breathlessness. I had a fever, aches, and extreme fatigue as well.

I knew from my Buteyko training that if I tried to take bigger breaths when breathless, it would only lead to more difficulty. The principle of Buteyko Breathing Education is not to over-breathe but to keep your breathing quiet and relaxed. And I kept nasal-breathing even though I was tempted to open my mouth and grab for more air. A single mouth breath would make me breathless, while calming my breathing relaxed the coughing and kept my nose from getting stuffed.

Most important was knowing and being able to feel the anatomical pathway of the breath traveling into my lungs and back out. Having the anatomical knowledge presented in this chapter was instrumental in my recovery. Knowing the pathway that breath would take allowed me to focus my attention and be mindful of the *sensation* of the air as it traveled.

I knew I was breathing. I knew that the air was reaching my lungs. I could feel my body being touched by breath. I practiced *Sa~Ha* meditation to allow my lungs to bring in the air and reduce my willful efforting. All of this felt soothing and moved me from the panic of *I can't get enough air* to *My body is breathing. I can feel it moving in and out.*

The quieter and more observant I became, the easier it was to find air and allow it to nourish me, and I was able to keep the asthma at bay. In moments when it became more difficult, I used Hyperventilation-Reduction Exercise #1 (see Appendix D), taking the count to 10 and back. The few times I needed to do that, it settled my breathing right away, including once in the middle of the night, after which I was able to go back to sleep.

I could tell it was working, because I didn't feel breathless. And I could feel the response of my body. Rather than only breathing with a tight chest, I was able to sense the movement of breath in the back of my lungs and the movement of the diaphragm, maximizing the capacity of my breath to nourish me and keeping my mind still and out of anxiety.

As air enters our nostrils, it encounters three small bones on each side that *spiral* the air inside our nose and sinuses until it's conditioned to move down the throat to the trachea (windpipe), and from there it branches into two tubes (bronchi) that carry breath into the lungs. The branches of the lungs are like the branches of a tree. A tree's branches are a living extension of the trunk, receiving nourishment drawn up from the roots. The mycelium network beneath the earth connects each tree to the community of trees, spreading information and delivering support to each one, and allowing the stronger trees to support those that need extra nutrients.

In a similar way, the branches of the lungs shunt air from one part to another, wherever the air of breath is needed, all in concert for the well-being of the whole—a branching network that supports the whole organism. We take in the sustenance of the oxygen, which was produced by the photosynthesis of the leaves of trees and plants, fed to the cells and then breathed out to once again feed the trees and plants. All of this is powered by sunlight, feeding light to the trees to ignite the spark and fire within, to bring life to all realms of being. The best thing I could do for myself in my time of COVID was to lie in the sun for a short period each day, receiving vitamin D and the heat and light of its rays.

I was invited to teach Continuum in Stockholm and share my knowledge of breathing. Stockholm is a wonderful city of many small islands and a mainland surrounded by water, with wonderful reflected light. Each group who attended my classes was enthusiastic, and in spite of my not being able to speak Swedish, the language of the body was easily transmitted.

On days when the sun was shining, even though the temperature didn't rise above 65 degrees F, the parks were filled with people in various stages of undress taking in the sun and the smells of warm air deep into their lungs. They knew intuitively that the heat of the sun would benefit their health—restoring their vitality after a long winter's night. Breath's pathways from the tip of the nose to the deep recesses of the tiny air sacs of the lungs deliver nutrients from plants and trees kept alive by sun and rain. These passageways are our connection to all that thrives beyond the boundaries of our skin.

In recent years, forest bathing has become popular. Spending time in nature provides physical and emotional health benefits. No wonder! Both the trees and our human breathing are engaged in the same respiratory process. When we forest-bathe, we're in kinship with what we both need to sustain life. We feel the same resonance when we're by the sea. The inflow and outflow of the tides is very much like our own breathing process. The movement of the humid air arriving deep into the shores of our lungs returns back "to sea" on the exhale.

Envision the descriptions of the anatomy of respiration that follow in the context of this larger scale of community, and recognize the incredible complex structures within our bodies as no different from all other life, created to sustain existence.

Our lungs, like a large branching *bronchial tree*, bring in air to allow them to expand. The bronchial tree delivers breath to the alveoli, 300 million tiny air sacs wrapped in blood vessels. Capillaries pick up and store the oxygen in the red blood cell and deliver nourishment to each cell, where it moves to mitochondria, membrane-bound cell organelles that generate the energy that powers the body.

The by-products of aerobic cellular respiration are carbon dioxide and water, most of which are picked up by venules (small veins, like capillaries) and returned to the alveoli, while some remain in the blood and the rest are exhaled into the air outside. This cycle is repeated, on average, 20,000 times a day. We can become aware of our breathing by sensing how our bodies move as we inhale and exhale.

The respiratory system (like the digestive system) is open to the outside. It is lined with membranes that secrete mucus, which is a combination of water, carbohydrates, proteins, and lipids (fats). Mucus provides a protective coating for the sensitive airways. Immune cells (white blood cells) are carried in mucus. This is one of mucus's most important functions. The human body produces about two liters of mucus a day, and it moves debris out of the body via coughing, sneezing, nose blowing, or the digestive system. It's always better to let mucus leave your body; allow your nose to run rather than suck the mucus back in.

While mucus provides us with much-needed protection, it can be a bother if too much is secreted, blocking the airways and making it hard to nose-breathe. This is what is happening when you have a cold; the flu; allergies; asthma; or other lung-related diseases like bronchiectasis, COPD, emphysema, interstitial lung disease, cystic fibrosis, infection, or gastroesophageal reflux (GERD).

The air we inhale is right under our noses. When it enters the nose, it's called breath. When it leaves the body, it becomes air again. The nose is an empty space defined by the outside edges of the nasal cavity and some of the skull bones. There are a pair of bones at the top where glasses rest on the face. Below these bones, cartilage forms the shape of the nose, and skin covers it all. The internal part of the nose is called the vestibule, which contains the septum, separating the nasal cavity into two halves. The nose of each person is different in both outward appearance and internal structure. In some people, one half is larger than the other. These sizes and shapes determine the volume and flow of air through each nostril. Which nostril dominates breathing changes every 20 to 90 minutes, as discussed in Chapter 2.

Farther back in the nose, on each side are three small bones. Individually they are called *concha*, and each is covered by a mucous membrane. These structures are also called *turbinates*. Both terms, *concha* and *turbinate*, suggest the role these bones play in determining how the air flows. The turbinates spiral the air around the inside of the nasal cavity on its way through the sinuses. Spiraling allows the air to touch more of the inner surfaces of the nasal cavity.

The septum and turbinates provide internal definition. The septum separates the nasal cavity into left and right halves, and the turbinates further divide the nasal cavity into smaller regions. There is a superior (top), middle, and inferior (bottom) turbinate on each side. The shape of the bones creates the openings for the air to flow through. The turbinates can become swollen from allergies and other sources of inflammation, limiting the flow of air and causing air "hunger" and the desire to mouth-breathe. Swollen turbinates can be one of the obstructions in sleep apnea.

Each of these openings moves to stimulate different parts of the brain just like alternate-nostril breathing. The lower opening corresponds to the brain stem or reptilian response. The middle opening, the limbic or emotional response. The topmost opening stimulates thinking and bliss. Early in life we develop a style of breathing that limits the flow of air so it mostly moves through only one or two of the three openings.

The sinuses are a system of hollow cavities that condition the air as it passes through en route to the lungs. The largest sinus cavities are about an inch across, the others much smaller. Our nose and sinuses have around 30 functions; the primary one is to produce the mucus that protects the nose from pollutants, microorganisms, dust, and dirt and to help regulate the temperature of the incoming air.

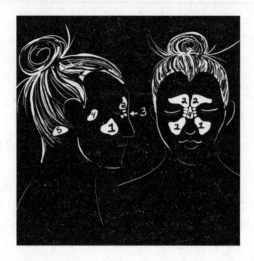

There are five pairs of sinuses in the head, connected to one another by narrow channels:

1. The *maxillary sinuses* are the largest. They're located on either side of the nose, in the cheek area under the eyes. Place your fingers there and breathe in and out a few times to feel for the movement of breath. This movement can be subtle, so touch lightly.

2. The *frontal sinuses* are above your eyebrows. Touch them lightly and breathe.

3. The *ethmoid sinuses* are a hollow space located on the sides of the bridge of your nose. Touch them and breathe. These might be more difficult to feel. Touching the area, whether or not you feel the movement, provides a sense of the territory of these sinuses.

4. The *sphenoid sinus* is behind the bridge of your nose. This is also difficult to sense as you place a finger or two there.

5. The *mastoid sinuses* are on the skull right behind the middle of each ear. Yes, air travels all the way

to the back of your head, helping keep it light and balanced. The bones of the mastoid sinuses are also the attachment sites for some of your back muscles that connect to your lower spine. You can feel them by placing a finger behind your ear at the level of your earlobe, at the bottommost portion of the skull in this location before you feel the neck.

The circulation of breath through the sinuses during childhood helps them grow and produce the mucus to lubricate the interior surfaces, preventing them from stagnating or becoming inflamed.

After breath passes through the nose and sinuses, it travels down the *pharynx* (back of the throat), through the *larynx* (voice box), and into the *trachea* (windpipe). The trachea responds to the flow of breath, so calling it a *pipe* may be misleading. We might picture it as a mechanical device, rather than the living, moving structure it is.

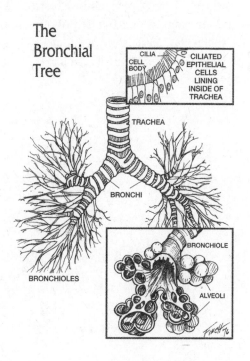

The
Bronchial
Tree

CILIA
CELL
BODY

CILIATED
EPITHELIAL
CELLS
LINING
INSIDE OF
TRACHEA

TRACHEA

BRONCHI

BRONCHIOLE

BRONCHIOLES

ALVEOLI

The trachea is divided into two *bronchial tubes*, which divide into smaller air passages called *bronchi* and then into a series of smaller tubes called *bronchioles*. These lead to the 300 million microscopic, elastic air sacs I've mentioned, the *alveoli*—the final destination of breath. Once again, imagine a tree and its branches, and you'll get an idea of the inside of the lungs. From our lungs, the oxygen of our inhale goes into our red blood cells. That process will be explained further in Chapter 8, "The Chemistry of Respiration."

If you put your finger in the notch at the top of your sternum (breastbone) and trace the sternum down for about an inch, you will come to a slight bump. That is approximately where the air enters your lungs through the bronchial tubes. The left lung has three lobes; the right has two. The average lung capacity is about 4.2 liters of air in women and 6 liters in men.

During normal, non-exertional breathing, we inhale and exhale about half a liter of air, which means we're refreshing about one-eighth in women and one-twelfth in men, respectively, of the air our lungs contain. During periods of exertion, we're likely to use some residual air beyond one-twelfth of a normal breath, and that cannot be sustained. Rest is required afterward to allow the lungs to restore their reserves to full capacity.

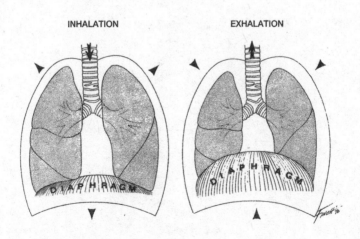

INHALATION   EXHALATION

Having our lungs "filled to capacity" is only possible when they're capable of inflating to their full size. For many people, their lungs are limited by the range of movement of their rib basket; the diaphragm; and the muscles, tendons, and connective tissues that move them. Breathing habits that arise from trauma, illness, or learned limiting beliefs contribute to this contraction as well, commonly in the ribs, belly, and chest, the very structures that need to be open and flexible for breath to enter our bodies with ease. (I prefer to say *rib basket* rather than *rib cage*, as I find it a less constricting image.)

When our respiration is not at full capacity, we may experience shortness of breath and/or labored breathing. The body is in distress; we can't get enough breath and thus we're fighting for our survival. One way to address any challenge to full-capacity breathing is to learn to *recruit* undamaged areas of the lungs, areas we don't usually use for breathing. Many of the explorations in this book can be helpful for this. Lying on your belly (prone position) can be the best position to give your lungs a chance to resume normal breathing.

I cannot emphasize enough that no two breaths are exactly alike. Each is stimulated by the specifics of our internal chemistry, which our nervous system reads to determine what is needed from the next breath. The quality of each breath is also dependent on our emotions. When we feel comfort, joy, and well-being, our breath will be easy and satisfying. When we feel fear or anxiety, our breath will probably be rapid and short, high in the chest. Stress can wear us out and lead to susceptibility to disease. An antidote is rest and relaxation, allowing the lungs and respiratory system to return to normal when we're not actually in danger.

The surface area of all the alveoli combined is approximately 50 to 75 square meters, which is a little less than half a tennis court. These surfaces pass the respiratory gases—nitrogen, oxygen, and carbon dioxide—from the lungs to the cells and eventually the mitochondria via the blood.

In the cells, oxygen moves to the mitochondria, the organelles that generate most of the chemical energy needed to power our biochemical reactions, called *cellular respiration*. One of the by-products of cellular respiration is carbon dioxide (CO_2), which is then carried in the blood back to the lungs. Some of it is exhaled, and some is used for other biological processes. (More about this in Chapter 8.)

The tubes of the trachea and most of the tubes in the lungs have rings of cartilage, similar to the cartilage of your outer ear and the sides of your nose, which keep the tubes from collapsing as air moves in and out. Feel your outer ear to get a sense of how hard and flexible cartilage can be. Where the cartilage ends, the tubes are wrapped in smooth muscles that dilate and contract them. These constitute the *terminal bronchi*. When they are too constricted, it becomes difficult to exhale, as is the case with asthma and COPD. This is what causes wheezing in asthma.

There are two categories of breathing muscles: primary and accessory. The *primary muscles* of breathing do most of the work. The *diaphragm* is the largest muscle of the respiratory system. It's shaped like a jellyfish or an open parachute, and it separates the lungs; heart; and other organs in the chest, neck, and head from the digestive, reproductive, and urinary organs in the belly. The diaphragm attaches to the upper lumbar vertebra in the back, to the front and sides of ribs 7 to 10, to the back of ribs 11 and 12, and to the cartilage at the lower end of the sternum.

Three layers of intercostal muscles (*costal* means "rib"; *intercostal* means "between the ribs") expand and contract the chest cavity. The *external* intercostals are primary muscles of breathing. They attach on the outside of the ribs, above and below, and lift the ribs and sternum on the inhale. The deepest, innermost intercostal attaches to the inside of the ribs from the rib above to the one below, and this layer aids in ordinary, passive exhaling. The *internal* intercostals attach between the edges of each rib above and below, and assist in forced exhalation.

The second category of muscles of breathing, the *accessory muscles*, help when we need a bigger breath. These are the upper trapezius, pectoralis major and minor, sternocleidomastoid, latissimus dorsi, serratus posterior superior, and scalenes, which are located in the neck and throat area. The scalenes connect to the upper ribs to help lift the rib basket and create more volume front to back when we take large breaths. This increase in lung size lifts the shoulders naturally, not vice versa.

The ribs are the bones of the chest that protect the lungs and heart. There are 12 on each side, and they are raised and lowered during each cycle of breath. The spine is where the ribs attach in the back. In the front, 10 ribs on each side attach to the sternum via cartilage. The bottom two are the floating ribs. They attach only to the spine, in the back.

The ways we take air into our bodies are based on muscular patterns we've developed over a lifetime to keep our organism safe and alive. Some of these breathing patterns not related to illness may have developed in response to trauma; feelings that weren't safe to "metabolize" at the time continue to pattern and constrict our breathing and movement. These habits protected us against actual threats, and now the patterns are hardwired into our nervous systems, even as the dangers have passed. Gael Rosewood, a Rolfing and Continuum teacher, calls this our *breathing signature*, the way we habitually bring air into and out of our body. To change this pattern, we need first to recognize that it isn't serving us any longer and that an alternative can help our breathing be more satisfying and nourishing. An important tool for repatterning our breathing signature is *Sa~Ha*.

This chapter is basic to understanding your breathable body. Please refer to it as you continue to explore your breathing and the pathways that each breath takes through the body. Understanding and feeling breath as an inner, living process also increases your capacity to regulate your nervous system with breathing as an ally. As I had to learn, the point is not to memorize each of the elements of anatomy but to feel it as a living, moving process that brings you home to yourself.

EXPLORATION

BREATH FOLLOWS AWARENESS

Philosopher and mystic Jiddu Krishnamurti wrote: "Life is the study of attention. Where your attention goes, your life follows."

Notice that each time you bring your awareness to a specific location of the body, the movement of breath there becomes apparent.

Now, bring your attention to any location (part/place/area) in your body. While maintaining awareness of your breathing, do you notice any subtle wavelike movements in the area of your attention? To assist, place your hands on the area of your attention. Can you feel your moving/breathing anatomy? As the air of breath moves in and out of your lungs and through your airways, it will expand and release as the lungs and airways change size.

Stay with one location until you feel interested in focusing on another place in the body. Choose places near and far from your lungs and see if you notice wavelike movements that rise and fall with each breath. These are nonlinear movements initiated by breathing that nourish body/mind/heart and show you impulses for movement you might not have noticed before.

CHAPTER SEVEN

POSTURES THAT SUPPORT BREATH

A good stance and posture reflect a proper state of mind.

— MORIHEI UESHIBA, FOUNDER OF AIKIDO

The practice of conscious breathing, of being *with breath* to maximize awareness and well-being, is usually most effective when we attend to the position of our body—how we sit; stand; lie down; place our lips, tongue, and teeth; and use our eyes. The ways we hold ourselves can increase awareness of how our body moves with breath. Please treat each of the postural descriptions in this chapter as *suggestions*, not rigid instructions. Don't force yourself into any of these positions; instead, allow your body to find its natural pose and then notice how you feel as you breathe.

I find that when I assume any of these positions, I am optimizing my body's ability to breathe and am able to discern when my breathing is well-regulated and when it needs help regaining its rhythm, indicating whether I'm receiving nourishment from the process of breathing. Please try using these postures while practicing the explorations in this book and whenever you feel that your breathing needs additional support.

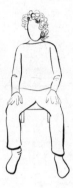

Sitting

Most chairs and couches are not designed for optimal breathing. They cause us to lean back, and when we curve our head and chest to look forward, our upper chest collapses over our belly, compressing the diaphragm, and we end up sitting on our coccyx, the tailbone. There are nerve endings in that part of the spine, and sitting that way compresses them and disrupts the flow of information through the spinal cord and nervous system. We humans are the only animals that sit on our tails. Other animals *extend* their tails as support, which helps them stand and sit in an upright fashion. When we sit this way, our whole body supports free movement of the lower part of the spine and eases the pressure on the diaphragm. We can describe this as the "horse-rider position."

1. Find a chair with a firm seat and a straight back,
    or place a cushion that's not too soft on the seat of
    your chair.

2. Move to the edge of the seat so that you're sitting
    on your sit bones—the hard, bony protuberances on
    each side of your bottom—with very little of your
    thighs in contact with the chair. If you're not familiar
    with your sit bones, try to find them with your hands
    as you sit.

3. Place your feet flat on the floor directly in front of you, a little more than shoulder width apart, the way you would on a saddle while riding a horse.

4. Let your hands drop down at your sides, which can help your shoulders relax. Or, alternatively, rest your palms (up or down) on your thighs, or place the palm of your right hand over your navel and the palm of your left hand on top of your right hand, with a very slight pressure so you can feel the movement of your belly extending slightly outward and back in as you inhale and exhale. You are not pushing your belly out or actively pulling it in.

5. While you're sitting in the horse-rider position, there should be little or no stress or effort keeping yourself upright and balanced. It is a *neutral position* for your body, meaning you're using very little energy to keep yourself upright, balanced, and settled.

6. You can follow these steps to help you find a neutral position:

    •   Lean forward a little until you feel the muscles of your legs engaging to stop you from falling forward.

    •   Lean back a little until you feel the muscles of your legs engaging to stop you from falling backward.

    •   Rock forward again, this time not as far; then do the same thing going backward. Each time you rock forward and back, decrease how far you go in each direction. Think of your upper body as a pendulum, with the arc getting smaller each time until you come to a pause and have no need to rock anymore as you feel settled "on top of" yourself. Repeat this as many times as needed until you get a keen sense of "neutral."

- Do the same from side to side until you arrive at neutral.

- To help feel your feet making real contact with the floor, rub them back and forth along the floor and wiggle your toes. If temperature permits, take your shoes and socks off for increased contact.

7. As the diaphragm (the primary breathing muscle) moves downward on the inhale, the belly moves outward. During the exhale, the diaphragm moves upward, and the belly moves inward. Don't force your belly in either direction. Just observe and see if this is happening naturally.

8. The horse-rider position is stable. Each segment of your spine has a round, bony structure, and each of these vertebrae is separated from the ones above and below it with a disc made of cartilage. Your weight is evenly distributed on these points: your sit bones on the chair and your two feet on the floor. Sitting in the horse-rider position, you are in your best approximation of being naturally erect, with your head on top of your spine without effort.[1]

9. Your eyes are looking about 10 degrees above the horizon. Try not to collapse your spine backward and lose its natural curve.

10. Breathe slowly through your nose (*Sa~Ha*) and feel for the breath low in your belly. While noticing the quality of your breathing, allow each exhale to soften your body and deepen your awareness of your contact with the support of the chair.

The horse-rider position frees the stomach and intestines so that they don't push up against the diaphragm. The diaphragm requires ample space for free movement. When it's crunched against the digestive organs, it can't move easily and the movement of air into the lungs is limited, leaving you feeling short of breath.

If you'd prefer to sit cross-legged on a meditation cushion on the floor, that too keeps the spine erect and the tailbone free. In most meditation positions, whether on a cushion or a chair, your tailbone is free behind you. On my office chair, I place a cushion that tilts me forward and has an opening in the back for my tailbone.

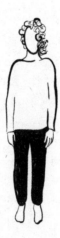

Standing and Walking

While standing or walking, we have a smaller surface beneath us than when we're sitting or lying down. We rely solely on our feet to contact the ground for support and keep us erect.

1. While standing (wearing shoes or barefoot), slide the bottoms of your feet forward and backward on the floor or ground. If you do not have the ability to stand or walk, practice this exploration in the seated or lying-down posture.

2. Next, pivot your feet while keeping your heels in one place.

3. Pivot again, keeping your toes in one place.

4. And finally, wiggle your toes and see if these movements provide more connection to the surface below you. We did a similar exploration in the horse-rider posture, leaning forward and backward, then from side to side, to help us find a neutral position.

5. Stand still and take a moment to appreciate your feet. You are asking them to carry your entire body weight all day long.

6. Notice whether you feel calm within as some of the tensions in your body ease. This too is "neutral."

7. Now take a baseline of the quality of your breathing and the capacity to get the kind of breath that satisfies. Practice *Sa~Ha* for a moment.

8. Walk around the room or outdoors slowly, while staying aware of your feet supporting you. If you lose awareness of the connection, stop for a moment and reconnect with your feet, and then begin walking again. Notice what happens to your breathing when you lose connection with your feet and the surface you're standing on, and what happens when you regain connection.

9. Anytime you notice that you're becoming anxious while sitting or standing and need to settle your nervous system and your breathing, reconnect to the earth's support through your feet. That can settle your breathing and settle your nervous system's response.

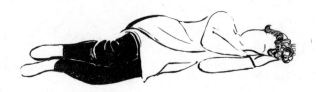

Lying on Your Side

1. Lie down on one side, then the other, and take a baseline of each to determine on which side you find it easier to breathe. This may be the best position for you while sleeping.

2. If needed, place a small pillow under your head. Be sure your neck doesn't bend too far forward because of a pillow that's too big, as you don't want to impede the spiral of air flowing through your throat into your lungs.

3. You can place another pillow between your knees, if you'd like, to make this position as comfortable as possible. You can even place your arms on a third pillow, or rest them in a way that feels comfortable to you, to minimize stress to your wrists, elbows, and shoulders.

4. Breathe in and out (*Sa~Ha*) in each position.

5. With each exhale, allow as much of your body to soften and make direct contact with the surface. The exhale is a time to rest before breathing in again.

6. Take a baseline after each position.

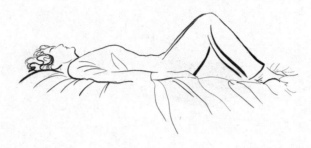

Lying on Your Back

1. While lying on your back, bend your knees so your feet are flat on the floor. (As an alternative, you can place your knees over a bolster, on a couple of pillows, or on a stack of folded blankets, or rest your lower legs on a couch or a chair.) This allows the organs below the lower ribs to move toward the pelvis and reduce any compression on the diaphragm. When your legs are straight (knees not bent), your lung capacity is reduced. Try all these variations to see if what I am suggesting is true for you.

2. Place your hands on your navel, using touch to feel which position—with legs straight or knees bent—is the least effortful.

3. Place a pillow under your head or a rolled-up towel under your neck, small enough so you aren't causing your head to bend too far forward and contract your throat or stress your neck. You want to be looking straight above you. When your head is arched too far backward and you're looking behind you rather than up at the ceiling, that can stress your neck too.

4. Now scan your body and notice all the places that your head, shoulders, back, pelvis, legs, and feet contact the floor beneath you.

5. As you exhale, release your body weight to rest more comfortably, feeling the support of the floor.

6. Take a baseline of your breathing.

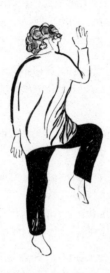

Lying on Your Belly: The Prone Position

For some people, lying on your belly will put a strain on your back and neck. But if the prone position works for you, it's a good posture to aid breathing when you're feeling breathless. In the early days of COVID-19, when there were severe cases and hospitals didn't have enough ventilators to support breathing, medical professionals put patients in this position, which they call *proning*. Lying on your belly compresses the front of the lungs, forcing air into the back of the lungs, where there is a larger capacity. Doctors would sometimes keep extreme COVID patients in this position for eight hours a day.

I read a news story about a man who came into the hospital with COVID-19 and only a 50 percent blood-oxygen saturation. Normal is 97 to 98 percent. They didn't have a ventilator available, so they put him in the prone position, and within a minute, his blood saturation was back to a lifesaving 97 percent.

Dr. Buteyko found proning to be the best position to prevent people from over-breathing. I find that it helps increase awareness of breath moving into my back, and by lying on my belly and doing it, I learn to access the back of my lungs. I also like it as it brings me into a calmer state. My most vulnerable organs are protected.

1. Lie down in a place that feels comfortable and supportive—on a mat, the floor, a massage table, or a bed.

2. If you'd like, place a pillow under your belly to ease the strain on your back.

3. Turn your head to the right or the left, or keep it straight by placing your head on your hands, on a small pillow (in such a way that the nose is free to breathe), or in the face cradle of a massage table.

4. To ease any strain on your legs and feet, you can place a small towel rolled into the shape of a tube under your ankles.

5. For an alternative position (illustrated above the title of this section):

    •   Lie prone with your head turned to the right (your ear directly on the surface or a small pillow), extend your right arm from your shoulder, and bend your right elbow 90 degrees, with your arm and palm flat on the surface, fingers pointing upward.

    •   Extend your right thigh outward from your right hip, and bend your knee 90 degrees, with the inside of your foot resting on the surface.

- Your left arm is resting on the surface along the left side of your body, and your left leg is resting on the surface straight down from your pelvis.

- You can reverse this position—head turned to the left, with left arm and legs raised and elbow and knee bent at right angles—to see which option suits you best.

6. Experiment with variations on these instructions to see if there is a way of lying on your belly that works for you, as it will be a great resource if you ever feel breathless.

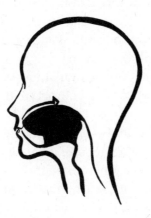

Tongue, Lips, and Teeth

The average length of a human tongue is three inches. Our tongue is largely responsible for our speaking, tasting, swallowing, and breathing. It is a wet structure that has eight muscles and 2,000 to 4,000 taste buds.[1]

Take a short baseline by noticing the position of your tongue, lips, and teeth, and the flow and effort in your breathing before you begin.

To begin, try placing your tongue on the roof of your mouth, its tip lightly touching the first ridge behind the back of your upper teeth, while your lips are lightly touching and your teeth are in close proximity, a few millimeters apart. Right behind your upper front teeth are a series of ridges. If you are unfamiliar with these structures, with clean hands feel for them with your index finger.

For some people, this isn't possible. The frenulum, the tissue that attaches the bottom of the tongue to the floor of the mouth, may not be long enough to allow the tongue to reach the roof of the mouth. This is sometimes called "tongue-tied." Some people have tongue ties on the sides that also limit the ability of the tongue to reach the roof of the mouth. For others, the mouth and upper teeth may be shaped in ways that don't allow space for the tongue to rest easily on the roof of the mouth. And for still others, their bite may prevent their lips from touching or their teeth from lining up.

If you're not able to place your tongue on the roof of your mouth, I strongly suggest you look for an orofacial myofunctional therapist in your area who can evaluate your tongue's movement ability; recommend procedures that might extend it; and provide exercises that can strengthen and maintain tongue, teeth, and lip positioning. Many orofacial myofunctional therapists and dentists are familiar with Buteyko Breathing.

Placing your tongue in this position, along with nose-breathing, facilitates the epiglottis lifting so that breath can flow easily down to the lungs. (The main function of the epiglottis, a flap of cartilage, is to cover the trachea while we're eating to prevent food from entering this airway.) When you hold your tongue, lips, and teeth in other positions or use your mouth to breathe, the epiglottis is less responsive, and its placement can hinder the flow of breath. Breathe mindfully (*Sa~Ha*) in this posture for three to four breaths while noticing the flow and effort of your nasal-breathing.

For comparison, try placing your tongue in the middle of your mouth, not touching the roof or the bottom, and see if you can feel how that affects the flow of your breathing. Then rest your tongue on the floor of your mouth. Sense and feel how these three positions affect the movement of breath down your throat. Which position provides the easiest pathway for breath? Most likely, your answer will be your tongue at the roof of your mouth. But don't strain to do this; remember that it isn't possible for everyone.

If you are able to, place your tongue on the roof of your mouth with the front tip directly behind your upper front teeth at the first ridge, while imagining your whole tongue as curved upward like the bowl of a spoon. The top of the tongue is meant to curl and lift upward so that it rests between the teeth on the left and right along the hard palate, all the way back to the soft palate. This may be more of an energetic feeling than an actual connection between tongue and palate.

In *Breath: The New Science of a Lost Art*, James Nestor writes that over the past 200 years, humans' mouths have become smaller and narrower. This can make it difficult to fit the tongue between the sides of the teeth and on the upper palate. The narrowing of the mouth actually lifts the upper palate and thus reduces the breathing space of the nose. Specialists in orofacial myofunctional therapy and dentists who specialize in airway function can help address these issues.

Your lips are lightly sealed, and your teeth are a few millimeters apart. This position of your tongue, lips, and teeth can help release tension and provide freedom of movement in the back of the skull and a softening of the shoulders, facilitating "nesting and resting." To get a feel for this lift of the tongue, try making the sound *Ack*, and feel the back of the tongue lifting.

The first time I tried this, my teeth began to chatter. I was so used to clenching my jaw, loosening the grip of protection felt threatening. Now, after a lot of practice and softening, and easing the tension in my throat and chest muscles (which I learned largely from *Sa~Ha* practice), they no longer chatter. This helps my face, tongue, and lips rest, and reduces resistance in nasal-breathing.

Bring this exploration to a close; then take another baseline of your awareness of the structures of your tongue, lips, and teeth and the flow and effort of breathing.

This way of holding your tongue, lips, and teeth may be different from what you're used to. Check and feel for any release and freedom of movement at the back or your head and the alignment of head and spine. You may also feel some additional core strength throughout your spine. Over time, as you find it more comfortable to hold your tongue, lips, and teeth in this way, it may become the natural placement for you.

Two related Continuum explorations that you can practice are in the section "Exploring Your Tongue, Lips, and Teeth" in Appendix G: "Hum Clock" and "Living in the Kiss."

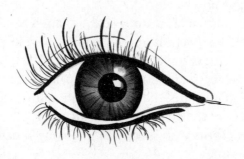

Eyes

Focal vision is when we narrow our focus to engage with what's right in front of us. We use focal vision to perceive details, patterns, and objects. Ambient, or peripheral, vision takes in all that's going on around us so we can make adjustments as we navigate our environment.

Since the pandemic and the increased use of computer conference software, time online, and activities such as video games and watching TV, people are spending more of their days in focal vision. Neurobiologist Andrew Huberman explains how this affects stress and breathing:

> [F]ocal vision activates the sympathetic nervous system [fight or flight]. All the neurons from your neck to the top of your pelvis get activated at once and deploy a bunch of transmitters and chemicals that make you feel agitated and want to move. . . .Vision and breathing are, without question, the fastest and most obvious ways to

control autonomic arousal. The way we breathe impacts our states of stress very strongly.[3]

Autonomic arousal triggers shallow breathing patterns, temporarily unbalancing the optimal biochemistry of breathing. When we're out in nature or just relaxing, our vision tends to be softer and more peripheral, gathering information from a wider scope of the environment. This is a practical way to know if we're safe. Animals in nature take in a very wide scope, enabling them to see subtle movement by predators or prey.

When using a computer, take eye breaks every so often and rest your eyes in a wider field. Gaze out at the horizon, with your eyes lifting to about 10 degrees. This can increase the ease of your inhale, and it invites a parasympathetic response and relaxed breathing. Activating peripheral vision can help increase a sense of presence and belonging in the immediate environment, while reminding your other senses to come online. I stay in peripheral vision as much as I can, especially while walking and working at the computer. When I do, my breathing is much more settled and deeper.

Go back and forth between focal and peripheral vision to see how they affect your breathing, the activation of your nervous system, and your ability to rest and settle.

CHAPTER EIGHT

THE CHEMISTRY OF RESPIRATION

*Over the oxygen supply of the body, carbon
dioxide spreads its protecting wings.*

— FRIEDRICH MIESCHER, SWISS PHYSICIAN AND BIOLOGIST, 1885

When the atmosphere, composed of mostly oxygen and nitrogen, is outside us, we call it *air*; when it enters the body, we call it *breath*. Like the wind, breath is an elemental force that spirals, undulates, and flows into and out of our bodies. The air you're breathing now creates wavelike movements that can help carry nutrients in and waste products out of your cells. This spiral wave returns to the atmosphere, becoming wind again. As you breathe in and out, you keep this movement alive and, in the process, come into harmony with the living universe.

Air enters the nose; passes through the sinuses; travels down the back of the throat, down the trachea, into the bronchi, and then into bronchioles, which end in tiny air sacs called alveoli, where oxygen is transferred into the blood vessels and from there into our red blood cells. There are five million red blood cells in each drop of blood, and inside every red blood cell are tiny protein molecules called *hemoglobin* (*hemo* meaning "blood," and *globin* meaning "protein"). Each red blood cell can bind to and transport up to 1.2 billion oxygen molecules.

After the lungs receive oxygen, it's transferred to the blood vessels that are wrapped around the alveoli and then carried to the heart. From there, blood is pumped through the body to provide oxygen to the cells of our tissues and organs. The blood circulatory system has approximately 60,000 to 100,000 miles of vessels, four times the circumference of the Earth. Oxygen moves in and out of cells by *diffusion*, the movement of molecules from an area of high concentration to an area with a lower concentration. When the oxygen supply in a cell is low, oxygen moves in to replenish the supply. After entering a cell, oxygen moves through the cytoplasm, the gelatinous liquid that fills the cell, until it arrives at small organelles (literally "little organs," *organelles* perform specific functions to keep a cell alive) called *mitochondria*, which produce chemical energy for the body's sustenance.

Depending on the function of a particular cell, there are more or fewer mitochondria. A liver cell, for example, contains between 1,000 and 2,000 mitochondria. Each mitochondrion uses one oxygen molecule; metabolizes (processes) it with other molecules, including glucose; and produces 38 molecules of energy, called adenosine triphosphate (ATP) and guanosine diphosphate (GDP) nucleotides. These energy molecules power other chemical processes of the body, including nerve transmission, muscle and brain activity, and organ functions, in a process known as *aerobic cellular respiration*.

The ancestors of today's mitochondria came into existence about 1.45 billion years ago, when the Earth's atmosphere was acidic and contained little or no oxygen. The only life-forms on the scene before oxygen and mitochondria appeared were anaerobic bacteria—bacteria that functioned in the absence of oxygen. Hence the *an*-aerobic, without oxygen. Mitochondria evolved from bacterial ancestors by learning to *use* oxygen, and now they're in a symbiotic relationship with us, living in our cells and instrumental to keeping us alive. Mitochondria can replicate on their own when there's a high need for energy and self-destruct when there's a low demand for energy. Mitochondria have their own

DNA, which is passed down through our mothers' gene pool from one generation to the next, and use a small percentage of our DNA in metabolizing oxygen.

Two of the by-products of the mitochondrial process of converting oxygen into energy (aerobic respiration) are carbon dioxide (CO_2) and water (H_2O). We exhale some of this CO_2 and H_2O, but not all of it. Carbon dioxide is an important ingredient of the chemicals that help to balance the pH (acid/base scale) of the blood. When our blood pH is balanced, oxygen flows freely from the blood to the mitochondria. When the pH balance becomes too alkaline due to over-breathing and a loss of CO_2, oxygen distribution to the cells slows down. Discovered in 1904, this is called the *Bohr effect*.

Carbon dioxide also plays a significant role in the body as a vasodilator. Vasodilation is the dilation (widening) of the diameter of the blood vessels for increased blood flow. CO_2 plays a role as a bronchodilator as well, widening the diameter of the airways for more air flow. Carbon dioxide supports the relaxation of the smooth muscles wrapped around the terminal bronchioles that might otherwise constrict and inhibit exhalations, as during asthma and COPD.

The levels of carbon dioxide in our bodies, not the levels of oxygen (except when breathing stops, as in sleep apnea), control how much we breathe in and out, and thus *CO_2 levels play an essential role in the health of our bodies.* Our bodies have sensors that track these levels in the blood and in our cerebrospinal fluid, the liquid around the brain and spinal cord.

The *Merck Manual* explains: "The brain regulates the amount of carbon dioxide that is exhaled by controlling the speed and depth of breathing (ventilation). The amount of carbon dioxide exhaled, and consequently the pH of the blood, increases as breathing becomes faster and deeper. By adjusting the speed and depth of breathing, the brain and lungs are able to regulate the blood pH minute by minute."[1] Dysfunctional breathing (discussed in Part III) can disrupt this balance and breathing behavior.

Another important benefit of nose-breathing takes place when the body is releasing carbon dioxide during the exhale. Two-thirds of that CO_2 remains in the sinuses at the end of the exhale so that when we begin the next inhale, we are breathing back our own carbon dioxide to maintain the proper levels in our system.

Imagine the dance of oxygen as it makes its journey from the atmosphere deep into the inner life of our cells and the return trip of carbon dioxide back into the atmosphere, a process that has been taking place for 1.45 billion years, feeding and nourishing the cellular life of our body.

EXPLORATION

MOVEMENT OF THE RIBS

Place one of your hands on the front of your chest so you are touching both the sternum and the ribs. Place your other hand on the side of your body. The ribs are meant to move upward and outward on the inhale, and downward and inward during the exhale. Feel for these movements as you breathe in and out. If your hand can reach your back, take a moment to feel the movement in that area. If not, do this exploration with a partner by gently placing your hands on their lower-back ribs as they breathe in and out. The ribs and muscles of breathing are meant to move in response to the lungs breathing (Sa~Ha). The rib movements support the filling and releasing of the breath.

Increasing your sensitivity to these movements takes practice. Trace the hardness of the bones—the ribs and the sternum—and the softness of the muscles between the ribs, and make a soft humming sound while touching these structures. Doing this can increase your awareness of them; and the more aware you are of your ribs, the better you'll be able sense how they move in response to breathing.

CHAPTER NINE

CONVERSATIONS WITH BREATH

True love is not a hide-and-seek game. In true love,
both lovers seek each other.

— MICHAEL BASSEY JOHNSON, NIGERIAN AUTHOR

One of the principles of Continuum is that movement is both the messenger and the message. As soon as I heard this, I could feel intuitively how breath too is a messenger, but I was not yet able to understand what its messages were.

So I paid attention, and over time I noticed that when I was anxious, my breathing was fragmented, quick, and shallow. When I was settled, my breath became soft, quiet, and deep. When I was depressed or lonely, I could hardly breathe. And when I was fearful or angry, I could feel the heat and fury of my exhales. I realized that these observations were teaching me the language of breath, that every mood, state, and movement—coherent or disordered— was reflected in my breathing.

So I began asking questions of my breathing. I'd been told over the years that I have a bad sense of timing, so I asked breath to teach me about timing. Then I observed how each new breath began, how long it took for the inhale to complete its journey, the time it took for me to exhale, and the length of the suspension between the exhale and the next inhale. Studying breath this way, I learned to go more slowly, to stop rushing. Breath finishes the inhale when it's ready, after it fully arrives in the body, and it departs from the body in its own time. I learned to be respectful and to allow breath to align with its own rhythms. And at the same time, I was learning about receptivity and intimacy. Forming a relationship with my own breathing taught me how I could be with others, how I could listen, receive, and connect.

Then I asked breath about receptivity, and I noticed the quality of my attention and the rhythm of my breathing. I asked breath, *How am I receiving you now?* Stop for a moment and ask that question and see the response of your breathable body. Receptivity, learning how to be receptive to your breath, can put you in a quiet, slowed-down state. When I'm receptive, the pace of my breathing changes—I give myself the time and the space to breathe.

I began to trust that breath is my ally. It's Mercury, the messenger of the gods, with winged feet, communicating deeply. I discovered that not only is my relationship with breath intimate; it is always honest. Breath reflects our inner state, and it's never distracted from delivering its message. It's a matter of listening. Breath follows awareness, and there is a triple helix of breath, body, and awareness inter-spiraling, intersecting at unlimited points and informing us of its insights, always responsive to new circumstances.

I decided to further explore the qualities of breath and the nature of intimacy. *Quality* is the degree of excellence, a distinctive attribute, possessed by someone or something. Qualities are features or characteristics of a person or a thing. *Intimacy* is the feeling of being emotionally connected and supported in something of a personal or private nature. Intimacy grows as you connect with someone over a period of time, and grow to care about each other and feel more comfortable during your time together.[1]

In my research I came across these five types of intimacy:

1. Emotional intimacy—cultivating a sense of closeness relating to how you and your partner feel via empathy, respect, and communication

2. Mental intimacy—a meeting of the minds

3. Spiritual intimacy—sharing a code of values or ethics

4. Physical intimacy—relaxing, joining in the flow, getting into the moment; it's all about connection, excitement, the giving and getting of pleasure, and closeness

5. Experiential intimacy—shared experiences; each of the other four types of intimacy includes experiential intimacy2

To achieve intimacy with others, I believe we have to know what is personal and private in us. We have to be intimate with ourselves before we can share intimacy or even be receptive to others.

Intimacy and receptivity require that vulnerability be present. A body-centered word for vulnerability is *permeability*, allowing information from the outside to affect our internal environment. And it goes both ways—exchanging what's inside us with the external world. This is the essence of communication and connection, and the essential nature of my conversations with breath.

We know how to regulate our permeability. We do it all the time—ingesting, digesting, and eliminating what's not useful. At a more conscious or voluntary level, we take our cues from others when it's safe to be vulnerable. We know when we feel safe immediately and are willing to trust. We feel open and relaxed, our body and mind are receptive, and even the pores of our skin dilate. In other relationships, trust and intimacy get established over time. And there are times when trust is never going to happen. The movement and touch of breathing carries with it an embodiment of all five types of intimacy. I knew when I first discovered somatic intelligence that if explorations with breath, body, and awareness were to be beneficial, they had to have a positive effect on my relationships with those I loved and cared for.

After asking my breath about timing, I watched and listened to my conversations. As a white male who reflexively speaks whenever I feel like it, I observed my habit of interrupting before the other person had finished expressing their thoughts and feelings. It became so obvious that it was like having cold water thrown in my face.

What other qualities are already in our relationship with breathing? Qualities like receptivity, connectedness, intimacy, gentleness, tenderness, fierceness, fright, anxiety, calm, joy, caring, excitement, love, tiredness, strength, weakness, sensuality, softness, and coherence—the full spectrum of emotions and feelings. Physical attributes like rhythm, volume, waves, spirals, flows, textures, completion, satisfaction, rising, and falling. The most profound of these are the qualities of connection and receptivity. Once we get a knack for observing breath, and it comes through practice, we can apply breath's teachings to the rest of our lives and to the health of body, mind, and spirit. In Appendix F there is a list of some qualities of breath that you may find useful to explore. We're building a vocabulary so we can speak directly with our own breathing body without the need for a translator. We're learning to speak the language of breath.

Once I learned to listen to my breathable body and observe its qualities, it became easier to follow its guidance and also the advice of Dr. Buteyko to go slowly, breathe less, finish the exhale, and allow breathing to be initiated by my own physiology, rather than its rhythm being manipulated by me.

EXPLORATION

BREATHING WITH FEELINGS AND EMOTIONS

Some people distinguish *feelings* from *emotions*, regarding emotions as impulses and feelings as the somatic response triggered by the emotion. Others define an emotion as a sensation with a story attached to it. This exploration gives us an experience of breathing with both emotions and the somatic responses.

As always, breathe with your nose. When feelings and emotions arise, breathing *with* them supports the ability to stay connected to their movement and appearance as they arrive and pass through. If you breathe out through your mouth when you're having a strong feeling, you dissipate the energy and disconnect from it. On the other hand, that can be a useful tool when you're unable to tolerate its intensity.

Bring to mind a situation when you felt happy. As the memory and feeling come into focus, nasal-breathe *with* it for a couple of breaths and notice if you stay connected to the feeling or memory. After those few breaths and one more inhale, with the memory still present, blow the air out through your mouth and see if the feeling or memory is still there.

When I have strong feelings or emotions and my breathing becomes a strong expression of them, I continue to nose-breathe as these feelings move through me. I want to know what I'm feeling, what is going on that's driving these emotions and feelings. Breathing *with* them, I receive an impression, after which I'm wiser and better informed. I trust that what I'm being given to observe is important. I also know that if it becomes too intense, I can dissipate the energy by mouth-breathing.

Neuroscientist Antonio Damasio tells the story of a man whose brain was damaged in an accident, and he lost connection with his emotions. After that, he was no longer able to make sense of his world or how to behave. Thinking was not enough. We need to know how we are *feeling* to function in the world.[3]

EXPLORATION

BREATHING *WITH* BREATH'S QUALITIES

Pick a quality of breath from the list in Appendix F or from your own experience. For example, let's use the quality of "connectedness." Say to yourself: *Breath, let me have a direct experience of feeling connected* or *Show me the quality of connectedness.* Then notice what comes into your awareness as you breathe *with* the concept of being connected to yourself. A question or statement like this invites the energy of that quality as you focus your awareness on *breathing with* and *being connected.*

As you go about your daily life, observe whether what you are learning about breath's qualities affects your relationship with others.

CHAPTER TEN

BUTEYKO BREATHING EDUCATION

The key to breathing that supports health is relaxation.

— KONSTANTIN BUTEYKO, M.D., FOUNDER OF
BUTEYKO BREATHING EDUCATION

Deep relaxation makes our body *breathable*. When our lungs are filling, our body is actually getting wider; and when our lungs are exhaling, we're getting narrower. Our whole body is responsive to the movement of breathing. When we're relaxed, breathing feels effortless.

But when we're holding tension anywhere in our body, that place cannot move freely, even to support the movement of air into and out of the lungs. In today's fast-paced world, it can be difficult to create the space to allow our bodies to rest and relax. As a result, for some people it takes a huge effort to breathe: "I always seem to be holding my breath" or "I'm often short of breath" or "I can't get enough air."

The Buteyko Breathing Education (BBE) method was developed in the 1950s by Konstantin Buteyko, M.D. Many breathing therapies help us calm our nervous systems, increase vagal tone, or enhance athletic performance. Buteyko Breathing Education impacts these areas, but primarily, in my experience, it helps us *cultivate a relationship with our breathable body*—learning which habits and behaviors serve functional breathing and which ones don't—providing us the ability to navigate our breathing body consciously and to self-regulate. Dr. Buteyko's goal was to help people return to a quiet respiration in harmony with the body's biochemistry, biomechanics, and psychophysiological processes, reducing the symptoms brought about by dysfunctional breathing.

Rosalba Courtney, an integrative breathing therapist in Australia, explains BBE's core teaching:

> The common perception is that the more we breathe, the better we live. Over 50 years ago, Dr. Buteyko observed, after many years of research, that the sicker people became, the larger volume of air they needed to breathe and that bringing the volume of their breathing back to normal led to elimination of their symptoms and control of their disease process. He then developed the following concept: *the more you breathe, the closer you are to death, while the less you breathe, the longer you will live.*
>
> To many people, this statement appears at first to be absurd and to go against basic intuitive knowledge. However, Dr. Buteyko developed a method of breathing based on training people to use a lesser volume of air effectively, which is one of the most potent means of correcting body physiology and eliminating disease that I have come across. In a short period of time, it dramatically affects the health of people with asthma, allergies, COPD, emphysema, anxiety, panic, high blood pressure, immune problems, sleep challenges, fatigue and stress-aggravated conditions.[1]

Both Buteyko Breathing Education and my training and experience as a breathing behavior analyst invite us to look behind the scenes of our breathing behaviors and notice whether the processes underlying the ways we breathe are supporting our health. Behind the curtain we see adaptations that we developed, some unconsciously, in response to traumas. We also see ways we think we are "supposed" to be and ways we think we are supposed to breathe. And we encounter the toll that air pollution takes on us, from secondhand smoke to fossil-fuel emissions and wildfire smoke. As we discover the many triggers of maladaptive breathing (which is actually adaptive to these unhealthy circumstances but maladaptive to long-term health), we also learn ways to mitigate adverse conditions and bring our breathable body into coherence, ease, and satisfaction as we receive and release breath.

The first study on the effectiveness of Dr. Buteyko's method on asthma was in 1968 at the Leningrad Institute of Pulmonology. The second, at the First Moscow Institute of Pediatric Diseases in 1980, led to implementation of the Buteyko method in the treatment of bronchial asthma throughout the Soviet Union. Since then, at least 17 clinical trials have affirmed the effectiveness of Dr. Buteyko's method.[2] At a trial in Brisbane, Australia, 20 patients who had long histories of asthma with significant medication usage decreased their use of rescue inhalers by 90 percent and of inhaled steroids by 50 percent, and their symptoms' score improved by 71 percent in just three months. Rescue inhalers dispense medication to relieve or stop the symptoms of an asthma attack.

BBE includes exercises for allergies, asthma, COPD, emphysema, pulmonary fibrosis, bronchiectasis, chronic bronchitis and pneumonia, breathlessness, shallow breathing, the habit of mouth-breathing, bad breath, dental decay, digestive challenges, fatigue, fibromyalgia, anxiety, panic disorder, snoring, sleep apnea, insomnia, athletic performance, and long COVID, and for children as young as four and adults with no age limit. These exercises focus on nasal-breathing, education about asthma medications, breath suspensions, and relaxation to help *restore natural patterns of breathing* that we unlearned during periods of stress.

* * *

I attended a Buteyko Breathing Education presentation in 2001 and knew immediately that BBE could help my daughter with her chronic and sometimes acute asthma. Then, a year later while I was teaching Continuum in England, one of the workshop participants asked what was on my wish list. I told her I wanted to travel to New Zealand and learn Buteyko to help my daughter and clients and to bring the information back to my Continuum community. She asked what it would take to do that. I told her, and immediately she wrote a check to cover the costs of the training. What a gift!

I believe to this day that learning Buteyko saved my daughter's life. I was teaching in Tucson when I received a call from her saying she was in the hospital with severe asthma and didn't think she was going to live through it. The mucus in her lungs had moved and blocked an airway, collapsing one lung during the time she was waiting for her husband to return home to take her to the hospital. Fortunately, he called 911. When paramedics arrived, she was passed out on the floor. They broke down the door to get to her.

I was on the first plane to her. I spent the next day teaching her the principles of Buteyko and practicing quieting her breathing, guiding her to feel the support beneath her body to help her relax, and two emergency exercises—Hyperventilation-Reduction Exercises #1 and #2, explained in Appendix D. She was a mouth breather, and I taught her to nose-breathe. The next day she was sent home, and she's been a nose breather ever since and rarely takes medication anymore. She can even laugh with ease now. Until then, whenever she felt an impulse to laugh, she'd reach for her rescue inhaler, as she knew that laughing would leave her breathless. She loves to laugh.

In 2003, I flew to New Zealand and studied Buteyko Breathing Education for a month with Jennifer Stark, one of the world's premier BBE trainers and author (with her husband, Russell Stark) of *The Carbon Dioxide Syndrome*. My good fortune continued, as I was the only student enrolled in the training and I had Jennifer all to myself for the whole month. During that time, we traveled to four cities to lead a five-day workshop at a hospital in each place. Each day, she would teach me over breakfast until about 10 A.M.; then we'd go to the local hospital to teach for an hour and a half. After the morning class, I'd spend the afternoon learning from Jennifer until 4 P.M., when she would teach another class at the hospital. At dinner and in the early evening, the lessons continued, as they did throughout the weekends. It was an immersive training.

Most of the class attendees were Māori, the indigenous people of Aotearoa (New Zealand), as the Māori have a high incidence of asthma. Our last series of classes was at a community center in New Plymouth, on the coast of New Zealand's North Island. Before each class, elders would *sing us into creation*, and at the end of each class, they would sing us out. This ritual imbued the class with a sacred quality, and Jennifer and I felt honored to be offering Buteyko teachings where they were so greatly needed and appreciated. One Māori woman walked five miles each morning to attend. At the final class, I was presented with a photograph of Mount Taranaki, the revered volcanic peak that represents belonging and strength,[3] and the image still hangs in my office.

I spent the next 11 months in Tucson, teaching classes on my own under Jennifer's supervision. I wrote a report on each participant, which she reviewed and offered feedback on. At the end of the yearlong training, I passed a comprehensive exam and became an authorized teacher through the Buteyko Institute of Breathing and Health in Australia. At the time, there were very few Buteyko teachers in the U.S. In 2010, I became a founding member of the Buteyko Breathing Educators Association in North America and a trainer of Buteyko educators. I continue to teach Buteyko Breathing Education classes internationally and in private sessions.

The guiding principle of Buteyko Breathing Education is to reduce the volume of breathing to achieve light and easy breathing that is soundless, peaceful, and restful; feels nourishing and satisfying; does not leave you wanting for more or always needing to take a deep breath; doesn't disturb your sleep, trigger other breathing-related conditions, or dysregulate your nervous system, creating anxiety and panic; and supports downregulating your nervous system into "rest, settle, and digest"—and to differentiate between over-breathing when at rest and losing your nose-breathing capacity and needing to slow down. All of this can be accomplished when you develop the habit of quiet, nasal-breathing and continue to nose-breathe through your activities. When you find yourself mouth-breathing, slow down and see if you can breathe through your nose. When you are able to *identify* a dysfunctional breathing habit, change becomes possible. Most people are surprised to realize how much they mouth-breathe and how much they over-breathe.

Many people, when they reduce their breathing from a pattern of over-breathing, find that breathing less makes them feel "hungry" for air, a natural result of inhaling less air than they are used to. This, of course, makes them slightly uncomfortable; learning to tolerate this slight discomfort of air hunger is like taking bitter medicine. They are learning that they can breathe with less air and still survive. This is especially important for people with asthma. When you are having an episode of asthma, learning how to slow your breathing and breathe less can be difficult, because the impulse is to grab for more air. But slowing your breathing and breathing less can help reduce the symptoms of the episode. As an asthmatic, I know this from experience, and for me it always works. Slowing breathing and reducing breathing volume *increases oxygenation* by retaining more CO_2, which helps dilate constricted airways. Studies of the Buteyko method have shown large reductions in symptoms and less need for rescue inhalers over the course of three months.

Recently, I e-mailed a flier to my list announcing an online Buteyko Breathing Education workshop, writing that I'd just had COVID and that without my knowledge of Buteyko and how to slow my breathing, reset and settle my nervous system, and find breathing space in my lungs, I might have been hospitalized. A former client e-mailed me back, sharing their story about a scary breathing event:

Last week, I was to undergo a "capsule endoscopy" procedure so that images that are out of the reach of a normal endoscopy could be gathered from the small intestine. The process requires swallowing a "small" encapsulated camera (about the size of the first knuckle and a half of my pinkie finger) and wearing some receiving equipment while the camera transmits data/imagery to it. Pretty advanced—if it works correctly!

I went into the doctor's office to swallow the pill, and it didn't go so well. I really thought I was going to be able to do it. When I tried to swallow the thing, it went sideways and got lodged on the right side of my throat where I don't have any muscle control (due to nerve damage). The pill was largely obstructing my breathing. I was using all the air I had left in my lungs to spit out words and say things to the nurses like, "I can't breathe!" (A nurse's retort was, "Yes, you can. You're still talking." That was not very comforting. LOL.)

It felt like if I really tried to take a forceful, big in-breath, the pill might go down my trachea. I didn't have enough air in my lungs to cough it out, and I felt like my air was running out.

I'm sure that the nurses would have reached down my throat to clear the obstruction, but I don't know how long it would have taken them to do that. I was panicked, and I guess that's why I didn't think of sticking my own fingers down my throat. . . .

All of a sudden I remembered your comment. I remembered it slightly incorrectly, and the words *finding small places to breathe into* came into my mind. I shifted my focus from *efforting to get breath* to just *slowing down my breathing*. I imagined I was sipping in breath through a tube about a quarter of the diameter of a drinking straw. I was able to take in enough air, slowly, that I coughed up the pill.

Over the span of four decades, Dr. Buteyko developed exercises to normalize breathing volume. In my work as a breathing educator, I focus on six of these: nose clearing; the mini-pause; restorative breathing (also called reduced breathing—reducing the volume caused by over-breathing); and Hyperventilation-Reduction Exercises #1, #2, and #3. Unlike the explorations throughout this book, these are *exercises*, meant to be followed to the letter, unless you simply must make adaptations.

Breathing is both voluntary and involuntary, and with attention and intelligence, you can guide the voluntary aspects of respiration by helping create a receptive field. How you receive breath can shift your breathing habits from patterns that no longer serve your health to those that bring long-lasting benefits. Deconstructing poor biomechanics, beliefs, and attitudes affects the chemistry of breathing and thus the intake demands of the body. Jennifer Stark teaches that the goal is not only to be able to *do* the practices but to *live* them—to incorporate quiet, easy breathing into our lives.

How do we know when we're being nourished by breath? What physical signs let us know that our breathing is supporting our basic needs and our overall sense of joy and satisfaction? One answer is that we feel a sense of *buoyancy* in our lungs from the fullness of each breath. When that's the case, appreciation, gratitude, and love flow through naturally. We feel more present and connected, responsive, interactive, engaged, open, receptive, loving, kind, and tender. Life's flow feels smoother. Our senses are alive; we're aware of sights, sounds, smells, tastes, and tactile sensations, appreciating the nourishment they can bring. We feel at ease, resourced, insightful, relaxed, and complete. Our immune system is stronger, and we feel *satisfied*, a job well done, breath by breath, supported by the earth beneath us, the space within and around us, and the breath flowing through us.

Relearning healthy, restorative breathing is a task worth doing. I offer breathing education, but your *breathable body* is your teacher. I can only offer suggestions based on my study and experience. I cannot—nor can anyone else—tell you how to breathe.

Once you experience your breathable body, its needs, and how to meet them, that knowledge is *in you*. Even when your mind forgets, your body knows how to receive air in "normal" times and in times of stress.

EXPLORATION

RESTORATIVE BREATHING: BREATHING WITH SUPPORT

This exploration is used in Buteyko Breathing Education to reduce the volume and pace of breaths per minute, to move from over-breathing to quiet, easy respiration, breathing that is allowed to find its natural rhythm without manipulation. (Please also see two related explorations in Appendix G: "Restorative Breathing" and "Feeling Support: You Have to Go Down to Go Up.")

In my experience, the best way to practice this exploration is while nose-breathing and lying on your back, your knees supported by a pillow or bent, your feet flat on the floor. This way more of your body is in contact with the surface beneath you. Once you get a feel for this, you can do it in any position, especially the horse-rider position (refer back to Chapter 7, "Postures That Support Breath"), which supports your breathing well. As you lie on a bed, a mat, or the ground, notice how your body meets the surface. Take a body scan of all those places to sense those connections and keep that awareness as you breathe in and out.

What happens to the inhale when you breathe with an awareness of support? Does it take less effort? Is there more space in you for breath to inhabit? More expansion? More capacity? Each time you breathe in, you may notice another area of support. Breathe *with* awareness of that support.

Notice if your body gets lighter as you inhale (buoyancy) and heavier as you exhale (gravity). Does lying there and breathing with awareness feel restorative or challenging, joyful or difficult? Practice this as often as you can—sitting, walking, lying down, anywhere you can rest your body—whenever you need support. The more you practice, the easier it will be for you to allow your body to receive the support it needs.

(For more information about Buteyko Breathing Education programs, practitioners, and resources, visit buteykoeducators.org.)

PART III

WORKING WITH BREATHING DISORDERS

Feelings come and go like clouds in a windy sky.
Conscious breathing is my anchor.

— THICH NHAT HANH, *STEPPING INTO FREEDOM*[1]

CHAPTER ELEVEN

DYSFUNCTIONAL BREATHING

Practicing regular, mindful breathing can be calming and energizing and can even help with stress-related health problems ranging from panic attacks to digestive disorders.

— ANDREW WEIL, M.D., AUTHOR AND PROFESSOR
OF INTEGRATIVE MEDICINE

When we were in our mother's womb, oxygen and carbon dioxide flowed through the blood in the placenta to our newly formed heart and then through our body. At the moment of birth, our lungs were not yet inflated, and they were filled with fluid. Around 10 seconds after delivery, we took our first breath, which sounded like a gasp, as our newborn central nervous system reacted to the sudden changes in temperature and environment. Following our first breath, which brought about an increase in oxygen in our lungs, there was a decrease in blood-flow resistance, and the fluids from our lungs drained or were absorbed by the respiratory system. Our lungs inflated and began working on their own, moving oxygen into our bloodstream as we breathed in and removing carbon dioxide as we breathed out. Our breathable body was awakened.

This first breath signaled a welcoming into the human family. We belonged. Each inhale reaffirmed this, and each exhale carried with it the fullness of life. Each human being is unique; you are the only person in the world like you. No one else can breathe for you. Breathing is your birthright.

Over time, in response to emotional and biomechanical misfortunes, our ability to breathe becomes compromised, and it takes its toll on our health. These acquired habits are sometimes called breathing-pattern disorders (BPD) or dysfunctional breathing (DB), defined as chronic or recurrent changes in the breathing pattern causing respiratory and nonrespiratory complaints that cannot be attributed to a specific diagnosis. BPDs are whole-person problems; dysfunctional breathing can destabilize mind, muscles, mood, and metabolism. They can play a part in premenstrual syndrome, chronic fatigue; neck, back, and pelvic pain; fibromyalgia; and aspects of anxiety and depression. It is estimated that 12 percent of the population suffers from dysfunctional breathing. Eighty-three percent of people with anxiety have dysfunctional breathing patterns.[1]

At some point in life, most people in today's world lose normal, balanced breathing patterns and begin to "under-breathe" (not take in enough air) or "over-breathe" (take in too much air). Both these tendencies result in biochemical imbalances that compromise our health, setting the stage for chronic diseases and a greatly reduced quality of life.

Imbalanced breathing is a hidden epidemic. Tens of millions of people suffer from health deficits brought about by dysfunctional breathing. These symptoms can be hard to diagnose and are often ascribed to other causes. Looking at breathing health first, in many cases, might save you money and bring peace of mind. It's time to focus on breathing behavioral patterns.

Symptoms that can be attributed to dysfunctional breathing include the inability to focus, brain fog, nausea, headaches, dizziness, tingling sensations, numbness, blurred vision, muscle cramping, increased airway resistance, air hunger, cardiac changes, hyperarousal, and reduced pain threshold. Dysfunctional breathing can lead to disturbed extracellular pH, dysregulated electrolyte balance, compromised blood flow and muscle function, autonomic nervous system disturbances, central nervous system deficits, and anatomical compromises or damage such as the misalignment of teeth.

These far-reaching impacts may—directly or indirectly—bring forth emotional (anxiety, anger), cognitive (attention, learning), behavioral (public speaking, test taking), and physical (pain, asthma) symptoms. Up to 60 percent of ambulance runs in major U.S. cities are the result of acute symptoms triggered by dysfunctional breathing habits.[2] Psychological effects may include heightened emotionality, anxiety, panic, disconnect, traumatic memories, attention deficit, learning impairment, changes in self-esteem, and even personality changes.

I use the word *dysfunctional* reluctantly. Dysfunction doesn't only mean that there is just one right way. Dysfunction implies that the needs of the person are not being met and that there's a more functional way. *Dysfunctional breathing* is a medical term for diagnostic purposes, but the medical model does not look behind the curtain to see what drives the dysfunction. Dysfunctional breathing presupposes there is a correct way to breathe, a proper way to behave. Rather than seeing the dysfunction as a problem to fix, we can look at breathing patterns as signals or messages pointing to what is driving those behaviors. Are they habits? Are they psychological, chemical, or mechanical? Breathing may express a body-mind patterned, perhaps, by trauma or unexamined beliefs about what is "right." Suppressing symptoms is covering over a gold mine or closing our eyes. Through inquiry, our breathing—whether "functional" or "dysfunctional"—becomes a tapestry telling the story of our life.

What is considered "dysfunctional" tells us that the current way of breathing is not optimal and is a starting point to bring attention to the possibilities of another way, that breathing and the body and psyche can be worked with, that having and knowing what is considered "dysfunctional" can be a stepping-stone for conscious change. To bring back the "natural rhythm of breathing" means to live with our own natural rhythms as the river follows its natural rhythms. In my experience, breathing is mutable, significantly affected by circumstances—as the butterfly in Peru I described in the Introduction taught me with an opening of its magnificent wings.

In other words, breathing habits can change. People who break free from old habits often report feeling that they have a new lease on life. They notice greater energy and feel more focused and productive. Many tell me they feel more alive and resilient than ever before. They invariably express surprise that such benefits can come about simply by changing their breathing habits.

A woman contacted me recently in desperate need of breathing support. She was emotionally distraught and could not stop hyperventilating. It turned out she was triggered by some neighbors who were illegally smoking in their apartment. The second- and thirdhand smoke was making her feel unsafe, which pulled up a string of traumas. Working with a naturopath and her therapist, she became aware of what was behind her dysfunctional breathing, and when she was able to express her feelings, her breathing returned to normal, allowing her to gain some perspective in her recovery process from the traumatic period.

We must each find our own way. It's easy to feel distraught, terrified, and at our wit's end when something as fundamental as breathing is not working well. In Chapter 13, "Asthma," I talk about the "fat folder" syndrome, where we go from doctor to doctor trying to get a handle on our distress. If we understand that dysfunctional breathing can be an important piece of a puzzle, we can try to become more conscious of the *habits* of breathing that produce these symptoms.

EXPLORATION

INTERVIEW CHECKLIST

To help you understand and learn more about your breathing patterns and under what circumstances, how often, and the ways in which your breathing might be dysfunctional, I'd suggest photocopying and filling out this Interview Checklist created by Peter Litchfield and Sandra Reamer of the Professional School of Behavioral Health Sciences. This list offers a view of the many symptoms that result from dysfunctional breathing and helps you refine under what conditions you may be dysregulating your breathing and having some of these symptoms. This list also helps you see how often certain symptoms appear.

INTERVIEW CHECKLIST
For learning about your breathing habits

This checklist has been designed to serve as a "guideline" for assisting you in exploring whether or not your breathing habits are consistent with optimal respiration, and if not, how they may be affecting you at specific times and places.

Name _____ Date_____ Email _____

Tel _____ Sex ____ Age ____ Sig other? ____ Children? ____ Issue_____

Do you think you might have a dysfunctional breathing habit? If so, what difficulties are you having that might be related to breathing?
_____
_____

Do you ever experience any of the 24 symptoms listed below? Check the **Y** column for "YES," OR the **N** column for "NO," after each symptom listed. If you checked YES, indicate *how frequently you experience the symptom* by checking a number 1 through 7, where 1 is rarely and 7 is daily. Then enter in the *situations in which you experience a symptom*, in the "situation column," by entering a number that corresponds to one of the 21 situations listed at the bottom of the page. For example, you might check column #6 for "dizziness" and then enter in situations #14 (expressing feelings) and #19 (learning new tasks). If the situation is not shown on the list, write it into the "comment" column. Focus on when, where, and with whom these symptoms may occur.

How often?   1 = rarely ....7 = every day

Do you experience the following? If so, how often?	N	Y	1	2	3	4	5	6	7	Situations	Comment
Chest tightness, pressure, or pain ●											
Intentional breathing, purposeful regulation											
Blurred or hazy vision											
Dizziness, light-headedness, fainting ●											
Disconnected, things seem distant											
Shortness of breath, difficulty breathing ●											
Tingling or numbness, e.g., fingers, lips ●											
Disoriented, confused											
Unable to breathe deeply ●											
Muscle pain, stiffness, e.g., hands, jaw, back											
Not exhaling completely, aborting the exhale ●											
Deep breathing, like during talking ●											
Fast or irregular heartbeat											
Chest breathing, effortful breathing ●											
Breath holding, irregular breathing											
Poor concentration, focus, memory											
Rapid breathing, panicky breathing ●											
Fatigue easily											
Worried about my breathing ●											
Mouth breathing ●											
Hard to swallow, nauseous											
Can't seem to get enough oxygen ●											
Hyper-aroused, can't calm down, anxious											
Unexpected mood changes (e.g., anger)											

*SITUATIONS: circumstances under which you experience the above symptoms

(1) working (employment)
(2) resting (between tasks)
(3) performing (e.g., test taking)
(4) talking, eating, singing
(5) feeling anxious or worried
(6) feeling tired or stressed
(7) interacting in groups

(08) physical challenges, exercising
(09) being confronted by others
(10) traveling, unfamiliar places
(11) socializing, meeting people
(12) speaking in public, in groups
(13) feeling angry or upset
(14) intimacy, expressing feelings

(15) physical discomfort, pain
(16) meeting authority figures
(17) going to sleep, while asleep
(18) being accountable, in-charge
(19) learning new tasks, new info
(20) feeling unsure of self
(21) allergens, weather, foods

General comments:_____
_____

Copyrighted 2014, Peter M. Litchfield, Ph.D. and Sandra Reamer, MFA
Emails: pl@breathingsciences.bp.edu and sr@bp.edu

EXPLORATION

Nijmegen Questionnaire

Another helpful checklist is the Nijmegen Questionnaire, developed by researchers at the Radboud University Nijmegen in the Netherlands in the 1980s as a screening tool to detect patients with hyperventilation complaints that could benefit from breathing regulation. The Nijmegen Questionnaire gives a broad view of symptoms associated with dysfunctional breathing patterns. It consists of 16 items to be answered on a 5-point scale ranging from "never," counted as 0, to "very often," counted as 4. The total score ranges from 0 to 64. Completing the questionnaire takes only a few minutes.

A score of over 19 denotes the presence of respiratory distress and dysfunction. The higher the score, the more distress is present. Values below 20 are considered normal and functional. Some say a score of over 23 suggests a diagnosis of hyperventilation syndrome.

The work is to become more conscious of the *habits* of breathing that produce these symptoms. If you discover from these questionnaires, the exercises and explorations in this book, and your own observations that you may have dysfunctional breathing patterns and symptoms, it would be advisable to check with a health-care practitioner specializing in breathing disorders and dysfunctional breathing. If you think you may have a breathing disease, seek medical advice. Visiting a doctor or other health-care practitioner in person, where they can see you breathing, provides an opportunity to delve more deeply into solutions.

Nijmegen Questionnaire

	NEVER 0	RARELY 1	SOMETIMES 2	OFTEN 3	VERY OFTEN 4
Chest pain					
Feeling tense					
Blurred vision					
Dizzy spells					
Feeling confused					
Faster or deeper breathing					
Short of breath					
Tight feelings in chest					
Bloated feeling in stomach					
Tingling fingers					
Unable to breathe deeply					
Stiff fingers or arms					
Tight feelings round mouth					
Cold hands or feet					
Palpitations					
Feeling of anxiety					

CHAPTER TWELVE

OVER-BREATHING

*Sometimes the most important thing in a whole day
is the rest taken between two deep breaths.*

— ETTY HILLESUM, DUTCH AUTHOR, 1942

The rest-and-settle response is an internal bodily experience. For a moment, we're emotionally at ease, and our "issues"—physical and psychological—are paused or even resolved. Everything in us feels soothed, in itself and in relation to all other interior parts. Our nervous system is balanced, and all other systems, particularly digestion and immunity, are functioning well. Our body is well supported by the ground beneath us and the space around us, and we feel expansive.

When something frightens us, our response is to take a big breath through our mouth. This is an instinctual and appropriate response. Adrenaline is released, activating the sympathetic branch of the autonomic nervous system, the fight-flight-freeze response. We either stay and fight, run like hell, or stand perfectly still to feign invisibility. This response to danger is meant to last only a few moments. *We eat the bear, or the bear eats us.*

Fight-flight-freeze is also an internal bodily experience. As with rest-and-settle, we still have the support of the ground beneath us and the space around us, but now we are *contained*. All systems are focused on survival, and all nonessential functions shut down so we can send extra blood and glucose to our muscles. Our circulatory system is pumping out hormones, and our nervous system is emitting impulses to sustain this activated state for as long as it can. All our mental activity is focused on the threat, and our vision narrows.

For all intents and purposes, this is the opposite of being rested and settled. These states are on opposite ends of a continuum, and for our benefit, we can move from rested and settled to fight, fight, or freeze in a fraction of a second. Unfortunately, going the opposite direction is a much longer process.

When we're in freeze mode, all systems are "frozen" to prevent visible movement. We're playing dead. Breathing is minuscule; bodily movement is either flaccid or tightly held. "Shush" is the operating instruction; *be quiet*. Nonetheless, this is a very activated state, and to come out of "freeze," we have to travel up the ladder of activation, which passes through the fight-or-flight stage. We froze from fear, and now we have to *process* our fear before we can return to being rested and settled, and it's not an easy journey. When people are repeatedly frightened, shutting down becomes the norm.

It's important to learn know how to self-regulate so we can return to being rested and settled and have that as our baseline. This means knowing ourselves, processing what keeps us activated, and being in relationship to our breathing and our internal experience.

Our autonomic nervous system controls our involuntary actions, such as heartbeat, the widening and narrowing of blood vessels, and the pace and rhythm of our breathing.[1] The autonomic nervous system has two branches:

1. Parasympathetic—rest, settle, and digest
2. Sympathetic—fight, flight, freeze, or collapse

These two branches work together, activating what needs to be stimulated to keep things running smoothly. The body rests and settles when it's safe to do so, and at those times it is easy to digest. When we're activated into a state of fight-or-flight for short-term survival, digestion—a nonessential process—shuts down so we can focus our energy on fighting or fleeing. These functions evolved so we could react when threatened and restore ourselves when not.

When triggered into fight-or-flight:

1. Our brain becomes more focused and alert.

2. Blood is diverted to the muscles, which makes us look pale.

3. Our breathing rate increases. Our nostrils and airways open wide to let in more air.

4. Our heart beats faster than normal.

5. Pulse rate and blood pressure go up.

6. Small airways in the lungs open wide to take in more oxygen.

7. We produce less saliva, and our mouth gets dry.

8. Sweating increases to cool the body.

9. Digestion slows down.

10. Our liver releases glucose to provide instant energy.

11. Our blood-clotting ability increases to reduce bleeding if we get injured.

12. The sphincter muscles in our bowel and bladder close.

13. Our overall immune response increases to prepare the body for protection.

With the evolutionary development of the neocortex, thoughts and imagination can also create a sense of danger. We're no longer limited to physically life-threatening situations. Our own nervous system may trigger the same fight-or-flight response as when a grizzly ambles by, and these kinds of activation can go on for a longer period than actual physical threats.

When we use our mouth to breathe, we trigger this activation and the responses listed above. When we use our nose to breathe,

the opposite is true. Nose-breathing supports a parasympathetic response of rest, settle, and digest. And when we use our mouth to breathe continually, we wear down our moving parts. It's exhausting and unhealthy.

EXPLORATION

FIGHT-OR-FLIGHT, REST-AND-SETTLE

Notice the difference between how your organism responds to breathing with your nose and with your mouth.

Place one hand on your chest and the other on your belly, and notice which hand moves first while you breathe in and out through your nose. Notice and evaluate the effort you're making as you breathe. Do you feel rested, settled, and at ease? What is your emotional state? Your mental-activity level?

Now notice these same things while you breathe in and out through your mouth. Which hand moves first? Notice the effort you're making as you breathe. Do you feel rested, settled, and at ease? What is your emotional state? Your mental-activity level?

Go back and forth between using your nose and your mouth to breathe, and continue to take note of the differences.

Almost everyone who tries this exploration reports that when they mouth-breathe, their chest moves first, they're making more effort as they breathe in, their thinking becomes more activated, and they feel less settled emotionally. And almost everyone reports that when they nose-breathe, their belly moves first, and they feel more settled. There are always a few who notice no difference or are more comfortable with mouth-breathing, perhaps because they are used to greater quantities of air. What did you notice?

Almost always, a fight-or-flight response triggers mouth-breathing. You need to get more air quickly, which is a plus when the bear is running toward you and you need to act immediately. If we do this only in extreme and real danger, the body knows how to return to rest-and-settle. But when we live in a world of danger—real or imagined—and continue to mouth-breathe, it takes its toll on our health.

When you are in a state of activation (fight-or-flight) followed by running, fighting, or otherwise mobilizing the body into action, cellular respiration increases, adrenaline is burned, and more oxygen is utilized to supply the energy needed. Problems arise when your nervous system is activated but then no physical exertion takes place. Your breathing and heart rate continue to be rapid, and it can be hard to catch your breath. You are *over-breathing*, also known as *hyperventilation*, what Dr. Buteyko called "hidden hyperventilation" because we don't know we're doing it until we have the symptoms.

Over-breathing can occur with trauma, stress, fearful thoughts, nightmares, allergies, asthma, lung diseases like COPD and emphysema, panic or anxiety, drug overdoses, COVID-19, severe pain, strong emotions, or just using the mouth to breathe.[2] Once I asked my son, who suffered from panic attacks, how he was feeling a couple of days after he'd told me he had an episode, and he responded, "What makes you think it's over?" His activation lasted for weeks, and I've heard similar reports from others.

Over-breathing upsets the chemical balance of respiration, reducing the amount of carbon dioxide and slowing down oxygen distribution, especially to the brain, and can leave you light-headed and dizzy, with brain fog, or feeling breathless, as though you can't get enough air and are unable to slow down your breathing or heart rate. When it becomes bad enough, fainting can ensue. Fainting puts an end to over-breathing and creates time for breathing to normalize. A folk remedy to increase levels of carbon dioxide after hyperventilation is to breathe in and out of a paper bag. This way you are breathing back your own CO_2, facilitating the release of oxygen to the brain and other parts of the body so they come back online and recover from the feelings of fainting. This remedy exemplifies the importance of the proper balance of carbon dioxide. (See the explanation of CO_2 as a regulator of oxygen levels in the body, known as the Bohr effect, in Chapter 8, "The Chemistry of Respiration.")

Over the years my clients have told me the kinds of situations during which hyperventilation happens, and three of the most common are driving a car, watching TV, and getting ready to go on vacation. Of course, many kinds of situations unconsciously remind us of something painful or dangerous from the past and trigger an activated state. I tell my clients to pull off the road and run around the car for a while if they have a panic attack while driving. Stay physically active until you feel settled. Exercise helps bring the body back into balance. The same is true if you wake up in the middle of the night in activation mode and can't settle down or get back to sleep. It doesn't have to be strenuous exercise; a walk around the house should serve the purpose. It can take hours for the adrenaline to leave the body.

Symptoms Associated with Hyperventilation

Respiratory System

- Upper-chest breathing, shortness of breath, chest tightness or pain not related to heart
- Oversensitivity of airways, excessive sneezing or mucus production
- Long-term blocked or running sinus, excessive yawning or sighing
- Spasms of the smooth muscle wrapped around airways, making breathing difficult
- Low carbon-dioxide levels, resulting in less oxygen released by red blood cells to tissues

- Poor sleep patterns, breathing-disordered sleep, restless legs, snoring
- Air hunger—constantly needing to take a deep breath
- Allergies
- Frequently licking one's lips
- Grabbing for air between sentences

Nervous System

- Light-headedness; headaches; dizziness; unsteadiness; poor concentration; numbness, tingling, or coldness, especially in the fingers, hands, or face
- In severe cases, loss of memory or loss of consciousness
- Increased sensitivity to pain, light, and sound
- Production of extra histamine, causing itching, eczema, hives, psoriasis, swelling, redness
- Blurred vision
- Chronic fatigue or exhaustion

Heart and Circulatory System

- Fast, erratic, or pounding heart rate, causing worry about health and life expectancy; palpitations; angina; arrhythmias; tachycardia
- Spasm of the smooth muscle wrapped around blood vessels, keeping blood pressure high and reducing blood flow to the brain and other body parts
- Increase in blood clotting, which may lead to strokes in extreme cases

Digestive and Urinary Systems

- Stomach bloating, constipation, dry mouth, belching, diarrhea, flatulence, irritable bowel syndrome
- Increased urination in order to maintain ionic (chemical) balance of the blood by the kidneys

Muscles and Bones

- Stiff and painful shoulders
- Stiff and painful neck
- Sore, tight chest
- Increase in lactic-acid production, causing muscles to become tense, tired, and sore, with possible twitching and tetany (a condition marked by intermittent muscular spasms)

Psychology

- Overactive brain
- Anxiety, depression, brain fog, nervousness[3]

When hyperventilation becomes chronic, people may have a wide range of symptoms. A patient may be sent to one specialist after another to try to find out what's causing the problem. Claude Lum, a respiratory physician in the U.K., called this the "fat folder" syndrome, describing the tortuous doctor-to-doctor path taken by many individuals pursuing relief from hyperventilation, during which their medical folders got fatter and fatter. Over-breathing, or hyperventilation syndrome, can indicate other causes, not just the way you breathe. There may, for example, be something wrong with your heart. If this is of concern, please have it checked out.[4]

CHAPTER THIRTEEN

ASTHMA

You will never know just how much you value
your breath until you can't breathe.

— UNKNOWN

During an asthma attack, the airways suddenly narrow, resulting in chest tightness, shortness of breath, coughing into breathlessness, and wheezing. Asthma leaves us gasping for air. One in every thirteen Americans has asthma, and the incidence of death and illness due to asthma is disproportionately greater among low-income populations, minorities, and children in inner cities. African Americans are three times more likely to die from asthma than whites,[1] and there are similar trends in Africa, Latin America, and Asia. According to the World Health Organization, asthma affected around 262 million people in 2019 and caused 455,000 deaths.[2] Scientists suspect that air pollution—especially secondhand smoke—is largely to blame. Asthmatics are "warning" us that our planet is becoming less habitable because the air is increasingly unbreathable. Factors like weight and diet increase the risk of asthma too, but the most overlooked factor is *the way we breathe* on a day-to-day basis. Asthma can be exacerbated by poor breathing habits.

As a child, I had coughing fits and would come up short of breath. That was in the 1940s and '50s, and asthma was thought to be psychosomatic (or at least that's what my father thought). When I was in my early 40s, I again developed a severe cough and found myself running out of breath. Whenever I was up in the mountains delivering papers, though, I felt much better. I guessed that the olive trees in the valley might be triggering my breathing problems, so I cut down the olive tree in our yard, and that seemed to help. Since the mid-1980s, it has been illegal to plant olive trees in Pima County, Arizona, where I lived, because of their pollens. Coincidentally, this often happened around my birthday, and I know there was an emotional component at that time that triggered my reactions as well.

It was not until I studied Buteyko with Jennifer Stark that I learned that what I had was cough-variant asthma, coughing myself into breathlessness and not being able to breathe. I also learned that many asthmatics have stronger smooth muscles that wrap around the airways, making breathing difficult, and more mast cells that produce histamines, which add to the inflammation response and increase susceptibility to a wide variety of triggers, including:

- Weather and atmospheric conditions, such as humidity, cold, dryness, heat, fossil-fuel pollutants, microplastics, wind, pollens, wildfire smoke, dust mites, and animal dander

- Colds, chest infections, pain, and illness of any kind

- Stresses and upsets that are beyond our ability to manage

- Foods such as seafood, chocolate, alcohol, dairy, certain fruits, and gluten

- Household chemicals such as secondhand tobacco smoke, cleaning products, incense, perfumes, and paint products

- Laughing, crying, exercise, and talking

If you have allergies or difficulty breathing, I'm sure you can add to this list. Physical and emotional triggers specific to each of us can result in difficulty breathing. Knowing your triggers is the first step toward establishing healthy breathing rhythms—quiet, unlabored breathing that matches your activity level and also originates from low in the belly and uses the primary respiratory muscles of the diaphragm and the external intercostals (the muscles between the ribs) to guide breath in and out of your body and cells.

When you can, it may be advisable to remove yourself from the vicinity of conditions that trigger your asthma, but that may be easier said than done if the triggers are part of your relationships or the atmosphere of home or work. *Even more effective than avoiding triggers is changing breathing habits.* Asthmatics tend to breathe two to three times faster than the medical profession's suggested rate of 18 breaths per minute. Dr. Buteyko suggested 12 breaths were optimal. That's one breath every five seconds. I hope that practicing some of the explorations suggested in this book and availing yourself of other resources will contribute to more ease in breathing.

Please note (*this is important*): If you are actively having asthma symptoms and are currently on medications, nothing in this book is meant to be a replacement for medical care. As you learn to breathe to meet your metabolic needs, slowly and deeply from within, and have a reduction in symptoms, you might want to talk to your doctor about reducing some of your medications.

Before I studied Buteyko in New Zealand and in preparation for being immersed in this field of breathing, I began to track the behavior of my breathing when I was having a bout of asthma: coughing uncontrollably, incredible terror at losing my breath, gasping and grasping, trying to relax and going to the mountains for cleaner air, using an inhaler. I was in a "state"—a state of anxiety and fear—the energy of the asthma state, struggling for breath.

Training with Jennifer Stark, I learned the science of respiration—the chemistry and its effects on my mental, emotional, and physical health. What a revelation! It made sense to me as an anatomy and physiology teacher and provided the motivation I needed to learn the principles and practices of Buteyko Breathing Education and apply them in my daily life. I wanted out of this loop of coughing into breathlessness and always being on alert for the next breath that would tell me I was heading into difficulty.

I was offered options to change my breathing behaviors and provide an alternative to the "state" of my cough-variant asthma:

- Quieting and slowing down the rate and volume of my breathing

- Becoming a fervent nose breather

- Placing and nesting my tongue on the roof of my mouth with my lips lightly sealed and teeth together

- Being careful that my postures supported breathing

- Deepening my experience of the ground of support beneath me

- Becoming aware of the relationship between the movement of my breath and my body's movement response

- Learning what it meant to finally find the state of rest-and-settle

- Inquiring into the emotional components of my childhood

- Applying the practices and principles of Buteyko Breathing Education and Continuum

The more I lived in these alternatives, the less frequently I had my asthma symptoms and the fewer "events" I experienced. Being able to distinguish between the "state" of asthma and the "state" of my healthy breathing made all the difference. As soon as I noticed one breath that was heading in the wrong direction, I could shift and breathe in a way that immediately reduced the chances of having an attack. I developed an intimate relationship with my breathable body and found that I could experience my entire body responding to the movement of my breathing. I was able to access a mindful state and apply it to my actions.

As I've mentioned, a severe asthma attack landed my daughter in the emergency room, where she nearly died. With her loving consent, I taught her about Buteyko Breathing, and we practiced quiet nose-breathing together in the hospital. She now credits Buteyko education with saving her life. She went on to practice the method dutifully for months, and she no longer suffers from breathlessness or asthma.

In 2007, I was watching *Dancing with the Stars* on TV, and Marie Osmond was the celebrity contestant. After she completed a samba with her dance partner, while waiting for the judges' scores, she was hyperventilating, gulping air through her mouth trying to catch her breath. Then, suddenly, she fainted. The cameras quickly cut away, and the network went to commercial. During an interview afterward, she said she had a history of asthma and had seen many doctors, but none could tell her why this continued to happen to her. She was describing her "fat folder," as I mentioned.

I found her e-mail address and wrote to her suggesting she try to breathe through her nose while dancing, and if she couldn't do that, then as soon as she stopped dancing, to close her mouth and nose-breathe to recover. I explained that by breathing quickly, with so much volume through her mouth, she was probably giving off too much carbon dioxide, and the oxygen supply to her brain was becoming depleted, causing her to faint. The next night the contest continued, and I saw her nose-breathing some while dancing and only nose-breathing while waiting for the judges' scores, and she didn't faint. I have no idea if she received my e-mail, but she certainly followed similar advice.

A teenager from San Diego and her mother, who was a nurse, came to see me as a breathing educator. The girl's asthma was so bad that she was often unable to go outside and spend time with her friends. Within just a few months of practicing the Buteyko exercises, she was able not only to go outdoors to hang out with her friends, but she joined a water polo team. Water polo is a strenuous sport. She was delighted.

Her mother also learned the exercises. Later she was at a soccer match when a boy around eight years old collapsed on the field. He was having an asthma attack, and he didn't have his inhaler. While everyone was waiting for the ambulance to arrive, the San Diego teenager's mother ran onto the field and took the boy through Hyperventilation-Reduction Exercise #2 (see Appendix D), which is a timed exercise that's difficult to do for yourself in the midst of an attack but is perfect to guide someone else through. She took this boy through the exercise, and when it was finished, his difficulties subsided, which may have saved his life.

When I was still in Tucson, a woman who was being hospitalized for asthma for two or three days every couple of weeks came to see me on her doctor's advice. After working together and learning the Buteyko practices, she was able to stay out of the hospital. Her doctor invited me to lecture at grand rounds, an educational program for residents, fellows, researchers, and others at the hospital. My next venture in the medical field was teaching for Dr. Andrew Weil's program for visiting doctors at the University of Arizona School of Integrative Medicine.

Buteyko Breathing Education has been useful for the thousands of asthmatics I've taught over the past 20 years—clients who'd had asthma since childhood and were now in their 40s, 50s, and 60s, and clients who developed asthma in their later years. Almost all of them experienced a reduction in symptoms, becoming less activated by their usual triggers and in some cases reducing medications under the supervision of a doctor.

To lose your breath is *terrifying*. Most asthmatics, myself included, can tell in one breath when breathing is going south. We're attuned to the pattern and quality of breathing. During an asthma episode, the first thing you do is grab for your inhaler while at the same time gasping and trying to get as much air in and out as possible. That's the way I dealt with my cough-variant asthma until I learned the principles and practices of Buteyko.

One time when I was in the Amazon, I had been free of symptoms for so many years that I no longer carried an inhaler. But something in the air had me breathless, perhaps smoke. I was terrified, being so far away from Western medical resources. Luckily, I had learned these skills. I kept myself quiet and practiced Hyperventilation-Reduction Exercise #1 (see Appendix D) over and over, each time I felt breathless. The exercise has long suspensions of breathing from the count of 2 all the way up to the count of 10, and then back to the count of 2. The suspension is not in seconds but whatever you are able to do. Each time I practiced this, suspending my breathing to the count of 10 was difficult. I had to develop a lot of trust that suspending my breathing would be effective in stopping my symptoms. On the way back from the count of 10, I could feel my airways relaxing and opening. Each time, the relief was astounding.

The suspensions were increasing my carbon-dioxide levels. As mentioned, CO_2 acts as a bronchodilator and shifts the blood's acid–base balance to allow oxygen to flow freely to the cells. That is exactly what was happening during my 10 days in the Amazon using this practice. I was diligent about nose-breathing at all times and pacing my activity levels to match my ability to nose-breathe. I took good care of myself and survived unscathed. As soon as I was out of the jungle, all these challenges receded. So it must have been something about the air quality. And I was fortunate because, as far as I could tell, it was an airway difficulty, not inflammation in my lungs.

In my training, I was taught that Dr. Buteyko believed that taking too much rescue inhaler and not enough steroids could be dangerous. If there is inflammation in the lungs, the rescue inhaler is not meant to have an effect on the mucus buildup. The steroids are meant to reduce the inflammation.

The mucus associated with the inflammation can move and block an airway, making it impossible to breathe. That's what happened to my daughter, and she almost died. Learning to slow down, breathe easily, and restore the balance of respiratory gases, allowing the airways to open and breath to flow, is the goal of Buteyko Breathing Education. Once accomplished, it can feel calming and deeply satisfying. Your breathing becomes your medicine. I'm not suggesting this is for everyone or even that practicing what you read in this book will end your use of an inhaler or your medications. By shifting to a slower breathing rate and less volume of air per minute, however, you are using your breathing to end your difficulty catching your breath. (For more information about Buteyko Breathing Education and learning these skills, you may want to contact a practitioner. Visit buteykoeducators.org.)

A WORD ABOUT "CLEANSING REACTIONS"

Buteyko exercises can bring up emotions, feelings, and symptoms associated with past illnesses. One time when I was teaching in Mexico City, the air quality was horrendous. I woke up in the middle of the night coughing with a barking sound, like someone with whooping cough, which I'd had when I was five years old. The tendrils (remnants) of this illness remained. Fortunately I didn't have to go to the hospital. I did my breathing practices and it cleared.

I learned that past illnesses that were suppressed with medications don't always "disappear" but sometimes go deeper into the body and remain undercover. Breathing practices that aim to bring the body back into health can reach into these places, so breathing can find its natural rhythm, without the energies of suppression that keep the body restricted. These are *cleansing reactions*. Try this exploration for slowing down your breathing and restoring a sense of ease.

EXPLORATION

REDUCING OVER-BREATHING DURING EXERCISE, ANXIETY, OR ASTHMA

When you are exercising and begin to feel breathless, this practice can help you quiet your breathing and build endurance. It can also be used when experiencing an episode of asthma or anxiety.

Don't stop walking at any time during this exercise. If the number of steps you take while suspending your breathing feels too difficult, stop holding your breath sooner, and start counting down to 3 or 4 sooner. You can always try again. Over time, your endurance may increase, and you may find it easier to exercise and nose-breathe at the same time.

- Breathe in and out through your nose twice, while walking. At the end of the second exhale, keep walking but suspend your breathing while you take 3 or 4 steps.

- Continue walking, and breathe in and out twice; then suspend your breathing as you continue walking for 6 or 7 steps.

- Continue walking, and breathe in and out twice; then suspend your breathing as you continue walking for 9 or 10 steps.

- Continue walking, and breathe in and out twice; then suspend your breathing as you continue walking for 11 or 12 steps.

- Continue walking, and breathe in and out twice; then suspend your breathing as you continue walking for 14 or 15 steps. In other words, walk and hold your breath for approximately 15 steps. If you have asthma, try to get to 20 steps.

When you reach the appropriate number of steps, continue walking while decreasing the number of steps until you return to 3 or 4 steps as outlined here.

- Continue walking, and breathe in and out twice; then suspend your breathing as you continue for 11 or 12 steps.

- Continue walking, and breathe in and out twice; then suspend your breathing as you continue walking for 9 or 10 steps.

- Continue walking, and breathe in and out twice; then suspend your breathing as you continue walking for 6 or 7 steps.

- Continue walking, and breathe in and out twice; then suspend your breathing as you continue walking for 3 or 4 steps.

Repeat as needed until you notice that your breathing has settled.

My wife, Nell, loves to ride her bicycle for exercise. She would often ride with a friend, who was a much faster bicyclist than she was. One time while her friend was away on vacation, Nell practiced a variation on this walking exercise. She counted each turn of the pedal as a step. When she became breathless, she'd slow down, practice this exercise, and then gradually pick up her pace while continuing to nose-breathe. When her friend returned, she was no longer able to keep up with Nell.

When I lived in Tucson, one morning I was walking my dogs along the river. About a mile into the walk, we came to a spot where they were building a new park. The night before they'd sprayed the area with jet fuel to keep the dust down, and when I got there, I started having an asthma attack. My lungs were closing down. I hadn't had asthma since I'd begun Buteyko, so I didn't have a rescue inhaler. I practiced this exercise immediately, and it worked perfectly as I moved away from the trigger (the fumes) while reopening my lungs.

CHAPTER FOURTEEN

BREATH HOLDING

*I wonder if Beethoven held his breath
the first time his fingers touched the keys
the same way a soldier holds his breath
the first time his finger clicks the trigger.*

— ANDREA GIBSON, POET AND ACTIVIST

When we're frightened by something, revisiting a traumatic event, or laser-focusing on a task, we might hold our breath. By "breath holding," I mean literally holding it, stopping breathing for a moment, or being so tense that we can only breathe into a small portion of our lungs. Doing this can help us not feel overwhelmed, but if we do it too often, breath holding can become a habit and we find ourselves breathing in fits and starts—a moment of not breathing, followed by a big inhale or a big exhale.

Unprocessed trauma is held in our tissues. As psychiatrist Bessel van der Kolk writes, "The body keeps the score." We buried these feelings at a time when they were overwhelming, and breath holding (also called "bracing") is an effective way of keeping these unmetabolized past events out of awareness. Holding our breath helps us avoid *feeling* unprocessed trauma.

Breath holding is a form of *resistance*. In electronics, resistors regulate the flow of electricity so as not to blow the circuits. The same principle applies in the body. Resistance is a useful strategy to protect us from becoming overwhelmed and dysregulated. I've heard many clients say, "I can't take a big breath. My chest is too tight." Their tightness may be a resistance, the body's attempt to slow down the flow of information that they might not be ready to receive.

I have learned to honor resistance and *breathe with* it. I see resistance as an opportunity to slow down and make my breathing volume smaller, allowing my body to swell gently with the inhale and to stop inhaling *the moment it meets the resistance*, usually expressed as tension in my chest. By meeting the resistance and not trying to push through it, I can invite the contraction to soften during the exhale. Breathing becomes easier and may reveal the story of a traumatic experience.

Breathing is an unfolding, living process. Noticing our breathing pattern can be a first step toward bringing about change, as I have said before. What underlies that pattern and might be driving it is, at first, unknown. Ask yourself questions like *What conditions are influencing my behavior, my mind and body? When, how, and where do they arise?* In the exploration at the end of this chapter, there is a list of questions you can ask yourself to home in on the biomechanics of the pattern as well as the emotional aspects that are conspiring to create resistance and how it might be loosened.

But we can't change patterns overnight. Change is incremental, and each step needs to be integrated before the next layer can be revealed. Remember therapist Matt Licata's counsel: "Safety first, exploration second, in a dance and dialogue and dialectic that will be unique for each of us. . . . Crafting a safe haven from which to enter into the tender places."[1] The work of staying present with our tender wounds is best done with the support of a therapist, a health-care professional, or another kind of mentor.

Most people who discuss their patterns of breath holding with me find it disturbing and don't understand why they do it or when it started. Years ago, I was demonstrating this process with a chest breather who couldn't relax his sternum (breastbone). Since the sternum is connected to the ribs, his whole rib basket was frozen. There was very little movement when he breathed. He was a man who rarely smiled, but as he allowed the tension to soften during the exhale, his sternum and ribs relaxed and out came a huge smile and a big laugh.

He remembered that when he was young, someone made fun of the way he looked when he laughed. One comment like that and he wouldn't allow himself to laugh in public again, a sad yet common story. He kept a tight muscular rein on any expression of joy. We humans are highly susceptible to criticism, and one comment can shut us down for a very long time. When resistance is honored and at the same time encouraged to relax its role of protector, freedom may be waiting on the other side. Breath may find a new expansion, which at first can feel strange, as we've become accustomed to constriction.

Ironically, breath holding demands *more* oxygen to provide the energy needed to maintain the tensional exertion. It's a vicious cycle: (1) we don't let in enough oxygen; (2) we're constricted; (3) we need more oxygen to maintain the resistance; (4) we're unable to expand for the larger breaths we need; (5) we breathe in through our mouth to get more oxygen ("over-breathing"), which may trigger the sympathetic nervous system and lead to anxiety or panic, which increases the tension, and on and on. We may feel as though we're suffocating.

Like over-breathing, breath holding affects the natural exchange of oxygen and cellular by-products. When we hold our breath, very little new oxygen enters our body, and after a while if we hold long enough, the O_2 in the red blood cells becomes depleted, lowering blood saturation levels. Carbon dioxide accumulates, which triggers an involuntary impulse to breathe again. The muscles in our diaphragm contract, forcing us to breathe.

You may think that over-breathing would bring in more oxygen, but when we take larger breaths over and over, carbon-dioxide levels in the blood lessen, leading to a reduction in oxygen delivery to the cells of the body. The delivery of oxygen from red blood cells to the rest of the body is regulated by carbon-dioxide levels and their effect on the pH of the blood. Over-breathing dissipates carbon dioxide and therefore reduces the flow of oxygen. This is called the Bohr effect.

By holding our breath after episodes of over-breathing, we slow the release of carbon dioxide. CO_2 levels rise, and oxygen once again moves freely around the body. Breath holding as an antidote to over-breathing sets up an erratic breathing pattern in which the body is always efforting to self-regulate. The body prefers stability, *homeostasis*, an equilibrium among interdependent physiological elements.

EXPLORATION

THE BREATHING CYCLE

Please stop reading for a moment and observe your breathing. As you inhale, is the movement of air a steady stream, or is it erratic? At the end of the inhale, is there a pause for even a fraction of a second, a moment of stopping and resting? Is the exhale a steady stream, or is the flow choppy? Do you stop before the exhale is complete? Is there a pause at the end of the exhale, or do you grab for the next breath? Dr. Buteyko said that a healthy breathing rate is 12 breaths a minute (one breath every five seconds).

Breath holding affects the sense of continuity in our life, of feeling settled in ourselves and in our body, the experience of one event flowing into another. Flow is the underlying feature of movement that brings us satisfaction and relaxation. There is an ongoing relationship of body and breath interacting with forces of gravity and levity, the felt sense of buoyancy and weight as the presence of breath shifts that experience, moment to moment. The feeling of our experience is intimately tied to the behavior of our breathing. Interrupting the flow of breath by breath holding interrupts the flow of life and creates a feeling of fragmentation, which affects everything, including how we walk, run, stand, sit, or lie down.

At the end of each exhale, there is a natural pause before the next inhale. Frequent breath holding does not give us time to land, to pause at the natural resting points in the cycle of breathing. Instead, allow breath to rise like a balloon drifting toward its peak and then gently, effortlessly, glide back to Earth and rest until the next current of air arrives to lift it once more.

Writing this book has been a demanding, albeit creative, process that provided lots of opportunities to hold my breath. As my friend Sharon Weil, who has been my greatest advocate in encouraging me to write a book, often tells me, "Resistance pops up everywhere. Don't wait for the inspiration to arrive. Just write, inspiration arrives when it does."

I take my sweet corgi, Nyx, on a walk most mornings at sunrise. We start out slowly and meander from bush to bush, Nyx stopping every few feet for another whiff. I'd go along with this for a while, and as my thoughts would turn to the book, I would start pulling on the leash and telling Nyx to hurry up. I noticed I was getting impatient. I love my dog. His innocent looks melt my heart. So when I saw myself being impatient with him, it broke my heart.

I noticed my shoulders were up to my ears, and I was breathing high up in my chest, holding my breathing small and shallow. That tight little space I created in my upper chest was all the breathing room I had. I was choking and getting more anxious by the moment. So I said to myself, *Find your ground, put your tongue at the roof of your mouth, close your mouth, breathe with your nose, and restore yourself.* And each time, it worked. Conscious breathing and embodiment helped me reconnect with myself, regulate my nervous system, and regain my patience.

These words came to me the other day: *One has to make room for breath*. The air of breath needs space to inhabit. It needs to fill our lungs and manifest the next moments of our lives, creating an internal environment that gratefully and gracefully receives and releases the flow. Breath can fill us up. A feast awaits us. We don't need to settle for meager servings of air that barely keep us alive. Whether we actually stop the flow of breath or whether our excess tension reduces breathing room, consequences and compensatory behaviors ensue. We "hold" our breath to keep it from nourishing our health, joy, and vitality. It's more than okay to stop breath holding; our life depends on it.

The average person will take more than 600 million breaths over the course of their life. Every breath stretches the lungs' tissues with each inhale and relaxes them with each exhale. The mere motions of breathing are known to influence vital functions of the lungs, including their development in babies, the production of air-exchange-enhancing fluid on their inner surfaces, and maintenance of healthy tissue structure. New research from the Wyss Institute at Harvard University shows that this constant pattern of stretching and relaxing also generates immune responses against invading viruses.[2]

It's time to breathe fully, to feel the rise and the fall of breath, knowing that it feeds us. When we do this, feeling the difference between healthy and constricted breathing, we will make peace with our fears and, at the same time, become actively intolerant of any context that limits our capacity to breathe. Over time, with concerted practice, many places of resistance in me have softened. Knowing these patterns and exploring them can open the doors of perception to what may be bothering us and causing us terror in daily life. Every day is new, and we can give our loving attention to whatever presents itself.

EXPLORATION

SITUATIONAL BREATH HOLDING

How we breathe changes with circumstances, as I discovered during my encounter with the beautiful butterfly in the Peruvian Amazon that I wrote about in the Introduction. Breathing accommodates where we are, what we're doing, who we're with, how we feel about ourselves, and the state of our health.

One evening after a long day of teaching, I was invited out to dinner by a group from the class. While I sat there, I noticed I was unable to breathe comfortably. I was too tired to be socializing. Rather than trying to be polite and stay, I knew it would be better to take care of myself, as indicated by my breathing. So I excused myself and went home, and my breathing settled. I often check in with my breathing, using what I know to make decisions and, when needed, to self-regulate. Self-regulation is managing our behavior from within through self-monitoring, self-evaluating, and self-reinforcement. Emotional self-regulation refers to the ability to manage disruptive emotions and impulses.[3]

As you become more familiar with the behaviors of your breathing, check with yourself and how you are breathing in different situations, such as work, play, or socializing with friends. Learning how your breathing behaves in various settings can inform you how to care for yourself by either changing the circumstance, responding differently, or using your breathing skill to self-regulate. Here is a list of questions you can ask yourself. (See also the Interview Questionnaire at the end of Chapter 11, "Dysfunctional Breathing.")

Situations and Timing of Breath Holding

1. Are you aware that you hold your breath occasionally?

2. Are there certain times of the day that you notice yourself

holding your breath more than others? Be as specific as you can. What activities might you be engaging in?

3. Are there certain physical situations that cause you to hold your breath?

4. What thoughts or concerns enter your mind just before you begin to hold your breath?

5. Are there particular images that trigger breath holding?

6. Are there sensations in your body that cause you to hold your breath when they arise?

7. Are there emotional situations—including feelings triggered by past memories or future fears—that have you holding your breath? Take time to notice if the situations are indeed current. Then inventory the following:

   • Past memories

   • Future worries

8. Is there any other reason why you might hold your breath?

9. Breath holding stops movement. What movement are you attempting to limit? Here are some choices:

   • Stopping any further input

   • Stopping movement to consider an idea and create a hyperfocus

   • Stopping movement to limit a sense of vulnerability that can sometimes accompany the exhale and resting at the bottom of the exhale

10. Are you holding your breath to get extra focus for problem-solving? To get a clearer picture of the problem and envision possible solutions, you freeze an image by holding your breath to get a longer look. This is not unusual when this need is present. I've noticed that when I do certain kinds of computer work requiring concentration and a new thought is forming, I might stop my inhale and use my mind's eye to see the thought and *then* start to breathe again. By sitting in the horse-rider position with my feet firmly on the floor as I type, I'm less likely to do this, and my thoughts flow more easily and completely.

11. How often do you find yourself holding your breath, and what clues told you that you were? Do you take a big gasp after holding your breath? Is that how you notice that you've been holding it?

Keeping a journal of the conditions and times during which you hold your breath can be useful in tracking down the behavioral habit and making a change.

EXPLORATION

BECOMING AWARE OF BREATH HOLDING

A Complete Cessation of Breathing

As you start to pay attention to the act of holding your breath, here are some inquiries about *where in the cycle of breathing you are holding your breath*. Knowing this will help you understand what function breath holding is performing, which is perhaps the underlying basis for the habit.

1. Do you hold your breath during the inhalation, and if so, is there a particular point in the cycle that you do so? At the beginning? The middle? Close to the end?

2. Do you hold your breath during the exhale, and if so, where in the sequence of breathing out do you do so?

3. Do you abort your exhale, ending it before it's complete?

4. Do you hold your breath at the end of the exhale before taking the next in-breath?

Take note of the posture and tensions in your body when breath holding is active, and answer these questions:

1.   What part of your body is being held tight as you stop breathing? As you are breathing?

2.   Sometimes you can become more aware of how and where you've been breath holding by noticing the moment and the location you begin to release the pressure of the holding. What is the next breath like after you have been holding the prior one?

3.   How do you feel after you release the breath hold?

Limiting the Size and Capacity of Breathing Due to Body Tensions: Holding the Breath Captive in a Tight Container

Once you notice that you're holding your breath, notice *how* you begin breathing again. Usually there's a grab for a big breath or a big exhale, often through the mouth, followed by a sigh. The sigh provides relief from the stress of holding. It's important to notice what you do when you begin the breathing process again after holding your breath.

As soon as you recognize that you've been holding your breath, gradually release the holding and start to breathe again slowly, through your nose. Avoid, if you can, gasping for the next breath or exhaling forcefully. If you must, allow yourself a larger breath while nasal-breathing to make up for any deficit of oxygen until the breathing rate settles down and the volume of breath is again commensurate with the needs of the body.

CHAPTER FIFTEEN

BREATHING-DISORDERED SLEEP

Sleep is the best meditation.

— THE DALAI LAMA

The importance of getting a good night's sleep cannot be over-emphasized. Breathing educators, doctors, dentists, mental health professionals, orofacial myofunctional therapists, naturopaths, and the many others who study sleep emphasize the grave importance of sleep hygiene on health. Phone apps have soothing meditations to help us get to sleep. Watches and other devices track our sleep.

Matthew Walker, director of the Center for Human Sleep Science at UC Berkeley, summarizes, "Sleep is perhaps the single most effective thing we can do each night and every day to reset the health of our brain and our body."[1] In his book *Why We Sleep*, Walker lists a phenomenal number of adverse consequences of not getting 7 to 9 hours of sleep a night, including a compromised immune system, certain forms of cancer, dementia, diabetes, cardiovascular disease, atrial fibrillation, stroke, depression, anxiety, suicidality, overeating, and even traffic accidents.[2]

In October 2022, I attended an online "Sleep Super Conference,"[3] and a few days later, I flew to Cancún, Mexico, to attend the fourth annual Breathing Wellness Conference organized by the Vivos Institue for dentists whose practices focus on sleep disorders.[4] At the conference, Matthew Walker illustrated the importance of sleep with these points:

- 24 percent increase in heart attacks when changing to Daylight Saving Time.

- We need to sleep before learning something, to be able to absorb the information. After learning, there is a need for sleep to keep it in our memory banks. We experience a 40 percent deficit in learning with a bad night's sleep.

- We have twice as much anxiety with insomnia.

- With poor sleep for one night, our immune system is compromised; there is a 70 percent drop in natural killer cells.

- There's an increase in cancer with night shift work. The World Health Organization considers night shift work a carcinogen.

- One week of sleep deprivation is enough to alter the activity of hundreds of human genes.[5]

- Poor sleep is a predictor of life span.

- Too little sleep significantly raises the risk of developing Alzheimer's disease.[6]

- Your chronotype, the natural inclination of your body to sleep at a certain time, is hardwired. To find out if you're a morning person or a late-night person, you can take the Morningness-Eveningness Questionnaire.[7] I am a moderately morning person with a score of 66.

All life begins with breath. Breath is prehistoric; our atmosphere is a circulation of all that was ever breathed and will ever be. Getting to sleep relies on our ability to breathe the air we share in ways that soothe our nervous systems and other organ functions to allow us to rest. Knowing how to take care of your breathing and your breathable body is a primary skill in getting a good night's sleep. If you are also practicing mindfulness, healthy nutrition, yoga, or meditation, or working with someone in orofacial myofunctional therapy, osteopathy, sleep medicine, sleep dentistry, or psychotherapy, conscious breathing can provide a baseline for you to evaluate how you are doing with these practices, all in service to getting a better night's sleep.

Virtually all factors that affect sleep hygiene are about breathing and how important it is to down-regulate and calm ourselves using breath. We need sleep so that our brains can process information, our immune systems can operate optimally, as well as a thousand other well-documented reasons. When breathing behaviors are dysfunctional—whether for mechanical, psychological, or chemical reasons—all systems are affected:

- The hormonal balance can be thrown off.

- The nervous system functions in ways that feel chaotic and anxious.

- Not enough oxygen goes to the brain and our mental activity gets destabilized.

- We can lose connection to our inner and outer worlds, feeling isolated and depressed.

- We lose our sense of wellness.

All these results of breathing dysfunction have deleterious effects on sleep, and thus on our body's systems over the long term.

Although there is no single solution to getting a good night's sleep, through breathing education, breathing behavior modifications, neuroscience, psychotherapy, somatic therapies, yoga, and mindfulness, we now have in our "toolkits" a multitude of ways that breathing can induce states of calm, and we can use breath as the first step in creating conditions for a soothing, peaceful, and calming inner life that welcomes sleep.

While we're asleep, our brain processes the information acquired during the day and renews itself by expelling waste products and creating a more balanced chemistry. Circadian cycles coordinate mechanisms that turn genes and cellular structures on and off. Sleep impacts memory, learning, mood, behavior, immunological responses, metabolism, hormone levels, digestion, and other physiological functions. One cannot overstate the value of sleep in maintaining a healthy brain and a healthy body.[8]

How long we need to sleep a night varies with age.[9]

4–12 months: 12–16 hours
1–2 years: 11–14 hours
3–5 years: 10–13 hours
6–12 years: 9–12 hours
13–18 years: 8–10 hours
Adults: 7 or more hours

Some 50 to 70 million Americans, or nearly one in five, have sleep disorders, including about 18 million who have sleep apnea, during which breathing stops for too long, lowering oxygen levels in the body.[10] When we have problems breathing during sleep—including apnea, insomnia, or snoring—health professionals call it *sleep-disordered breathing*. Roger Price, an integrative-medicine and functional-airway specialist, noted that it's not sleep that *disorders* breathing but the other way around. The way we breathe can disturb our sleep, and therefore it should be called "breathing-disordered sleep."

Although there are dozens of ways breathing disorders can affect our ability to get a good night's sleep, here are five examples: *hyperstimulation, sleep apnea, hypopnea, snoring, and insomnia.*

1. HYPERSTIMULATION

Hyperstimulation keeps breathing overactivated during the day, and that can carry into the night. We might fall asleep easily and then wake up four or five hours later, sometimes for the rest of the night. Consequences of sleep deprivation include brain fog, memory loss, dizziness, anxiety, exhaustion, restless legs, irritability, twitching, and breathlessness. Our digestive organs, heart, and lungs can also be affected. Before we try to go to sleep, it can be helpful to modulate and ease the stresses from the day's activities. At the end of this chapter are some explorations that can help with settling ourselves before going to bed or if we wake up during the night.

2. SLEEP APNEA

Sleep apnea is a potentially serious sleep disorder in which breathing repeatedly stops and starts. During an extreme apnea event, people stop breathing entirely for way too long.[11] If you snore loudly and feel tired even after a full night's sleep, I'd recommend seeing a specialist. In 2009 PubMed reported that obstructive sleep apnea affects approximately 20 percent of U.S. adults, of which 90 percent are undiagnosed.[12]

The three main types of sleep apnea are:

1. *Obstructive sleep apnea,* the more common form that occurs as a result of a blockage of the airway due to structural abnormalities, sleep positions, narrow airways, tongue size and position, and relaxation of the muscles of the airway

2. *Central sleep apnea,* which occurs when your brain doesn't send proper signals to the muscles that control breathing

3. *Complex sleep apnea syndrome*, also known as
treatment-emergent central sleep apnea, which occurs
when someone has both obstructive sleep apnea and
central sleep apnea

Here are five signs that might indicate obstructive sleep
apnea (OSA):[13]

1. Taking Middle-of-the-Night Bathroom Breaks—While
it's normal to wake up once or twice during the night
to urinate every once in a while, many patients report
going as many as six times in a single night.

2. Feeling Moody without Knowing Why—OSA could lead
to reorganization of brain's function causing irregular
mood regulation. Additionally, lack of sleep can cause
you to feel exhausted throughout the day, leading to
less patience, an inability to focus and irritability.

3. Waking with a Sore Throat, Dry Mouth, or Headaches—
The respiratory system can be irritated by OSA
symptoms, not only because of snoring but also
because many people with sleep disorders tend to
sleep with their mouths open.

4. Brain Fog—Cognitive impairment is one of the
most common signs of OSA. Memory loss, slower
reaction times, and impaired reasoning are just a
few indicators of affected cognition, all of which are
associated with OSA.

5. Feeling Excessively Tired Nearly Every Day—It is
normal to experience the occasional rush of daytime
fatigue; however, feeling constantly exhausted during
the day could be a sign of OSA or another sleep
disorder. Those who experience excessive daytime
sleepiness typically find themselves struggling to stay
awake throughout the day, often to the point that
they can't finish their work.

3. HYPOPNEA

Sleep apnea and hypopnea are closely related, and the two disorders share similar symptoms, risk factors, and outcomes. In apnea, breathing stops for dysfunctionally long periods. In hypopnea, breathing doesn't stop, but it's insufficient to meet the needs of the body, lowering blood oxygen levels, and if left untreated, can be a risk factor for hypertension, arrhythmias, obesity, heart attacks, heart cardiomyopathy (enlargement of the muscle tissue of the heart), and diabetes.

4. SNORING

Snoring is the hoarse or harsh sound created when air flows past relaxed tissues in your throat. Breathing heavily while sleeping pulls the relaxed airway together. As you breathe, the tissues vibrate.[14] You know the sound of the last sip of a milkshake through a straw? The straw collapses and you get little liquid but a big sound. This is like what happens with snoring. If you sleep alone, you might not even know you snore or have sleep-apnea symptoms. If you sleep next to someone, they'll probably let you know if you snore. Snoring can be challenging to relationships.[15]

Snoring is a common sleep problem. About 45 percent of people snore at least some of the time, and 25 percent snore regularly. In the U.S., about 37 million people are habitual snorers. There's a big difference between men (about 40 percent snore) and women (about 24 percent snore). Interestingly, only about 59 percent of snorers say that they snore. Snoring itself may not be a serious health problem, but it can be a sign of obstructive sleep apnea. Please review the symptoms of sleep apnea on page 150. Also, you can use the Snore Lab app to help track whether you're snoring and the dynamics of your snoring.

5. INSOMNIA

There are many subcategories of insomnia, which help health-care practitioners understand what is going on and how to recommend treatment. Generally, there are two types of insomnia. Short-term insomnia (also known as acute insomnia or adjustment insomnia) is usually caused by a stressful life event and lasts about three months or less. Chronic insomnia is a long-term pattern of difficulty sleeping. It, too, can be tied to stress, but it may also be related to irregular sleep schedules, poor sleep hygiene, persistent nightmares, mental health disorders, underlying physical or neurological problems, medications, having a bed partner, and certain other sleep disorders. Both types of insomnia affect both children and adults, and are more common in women than in men. Insomnia can arise during pregnancy as well as menopause.

In addition to short-term and chronic, a few other terms are used to describe insomnia. Sleep onset insomnia means difficulty falling asleep at the beginning of the night. Sleep maintenance insomnia describes an inability to stay asleep through the night. Early morning awakening insomnia involves waking up well before you want or plan to. Comorbid insomnia describes sleeping problems that are connected with a variety of other health issues. It's common for people to have overlapping sleeping problems. In addition, symptoms shift over time.[16]

I recently had an experience that revealed to me once again how intertwined breathing and sleep can be. I went to bed around 9 P.M. and awoke suddenly at 1 A.M. hyperventilating. I knew that in order to get to back to sleep, I'd have to bring my breathing into a quiet, restful, and soothing pace. So I practiced "simply noticing." I allowed whatever came to mind or body to be recognized—not resolved, just noted. I stayed present with what was demanding my attention. My only task was to be present for what was in my field, and to wait for sleep to return.

I *breathed with* each image, thought, and sensation that came into awareness, and doing so I was able to get myself deeply quiet, feeling the flow of breath become slow, easy, cool, settling, and nourishing. I was in connection with my body as it gained its full ability to breathe without restriction. I stopped hyperventilating by using *Sa~Ha* meditation, which also helped clear the stuffiness in my nose. *Sa* and *Ha* tuned me in to the movement of air being drawn in by my lungs, further slowing down the pace of inhalations and exhalations, and reducing the volume. I'm not saying it was a breeze. There were moments the voice within urged me to take a big breath, but I knew from many years of teaching and practicing Buteyko Breathing Education that breathing less would bring stability. Simply noticing my breathing, my thoughts, and my feelings informed me what I would need to do about what had been troubling me and, in part, keeping me awake. A few times, when rapid, effortful breathing returned, I practiced Hyperventilation-Reduction Exercise #1 (see Appendix D), and it quieted again.

I did this for nearly two hours, and when I began to feel sleepy again, I knew I had come to the end of what needed to be reflected upon that night. I went back into our bedroom, knowing that being with my wife would be co-regulating. If I had gone back to bed any earlier, my restlessness probably would have awakened her.

At the Sleep Super Conference, I listened to a conversation with Saundra Dalton-Smith, author of *Sacred Rest: Recover Your Life, Renew Your Energy, Restore You Sanity* and her outline of the seven types of rest we need for good sleep: mental, emotional, physical, spiritual, social, sensory, and creative.[17] And I realized that when I'm wound up mentally and emotionally how important it is to get the proper rest and feel nourished by a good night's sleep. So I began looking at all seven each day and asking myself if I was getting the proper rest in each of Dr. Dalton-Smith's categories.

For me, writing is creative rest. Swimming offers me sensory and physical rest. Quiet, mindful breathing offers sensory, spiritual, mental, and emotional rest. Walking my corgi in the woods offers me deep mental, emotional, spiritual, and sensory rest, as well as some social rest as I commune with the trees. Valuing my time with other swimmers, walking in town, Zooming and talking with friends, and evenings with my wife and corgi are restful social times. Occasionally nights out with friends are starting to come back after more than two years of pandemic isolation.

The question I'm left with is how do you find peaceful and restful sleep? Are you breathing in a way that feels nourishing and satisfying as it effortlessly glides through you? If not, what and where is your attention being drawn. What is on your mind that needs conversation and action? What is in your heart that needs expressing? Are you eating in a way that supports your breathing—things like not eating too close to bedtime or making sure you have enough energy to sustain your sleep and not wake up because your body needs nourishment? Are your hormones and biochemistry functioning properly and how might their behavior be tied to how you breathe? Are you having enough social, spiritual, sensory, physical, emotional, mental, and creative rest? What might be in the way of taking better care of yourself. How can you be more intimate with yourself and less fearful of self-discovery?

We are crippled by the pace of society, by the dominance of one class and race over another, and by the polarization of religion and politics. All these have an effect on the way we breathe and sleep. It is the context we breath in, and it sets the pace for short, fast breathing. Impressions fly by our eyes at lightning speed. Industrial sounds are pervasive and simply don't stop. How does an organism rest from all the input?

I have also taken to listening to music that lifts my spirits and opens my heart. This feels like spiritual rest.

GETTING A GOOD NIGHT'S SLEEP

Monitoring Your Sleep Position

Your sleep position is very important. As you age, the muscles of the airway lose some of their elasticity and tone. Sleeping on your back allows these muscles and your tongue to fall back into the airway. Your chin drops back, and your mouth opens and may be very dry in the morning.

Sleeping on your back can be the most comfortable position, especially if you have back problems. In this case, it would be best to put your legs over some pillows, keeping your knees slightly bent and allowing your belly organs to move toward your pelvis and away from impeding the diaphragm. (See Chapter 7, "Postures That Support Breath.") You can also put a pillow under the top of your shoulders and your head, raising your body to ameliorate the possibility of your jaw and tongue falling back into the airway. Putting small blocks under the head end of the bed frame is another way of raising your head while sleeping. Sleeping on your side, starting on your left side, is the better option. Or sleeping on your belly may be comforting.

Taping Your Mouth

If you wake up from a night's sleep with a dry mouth, you've most likely been mouth-breathing. Taping your mouth to prevent mouth-breathing probably sounds torturous and a bit odd, but it really helps break this habit and transition to nose-breathing. When you first try it at night, if it's too uncomfortable, take the tape off and retape the next night until you get used to it. I use hypoallergenic paper tape. It comes in different widths, from half an inch to an inch. For men with beards, I suggest using the half-inch width so the tape covers only your lips.

Step 1. Remove a strip of tape from the roll. Use a size that will serve the way you are planning on taping. (See step 4.)

Step 2. Immediately bend about a quarter of an inch at the end of the tape over itself, so there is a tab you can grab to remove the tape in the morning or during the night for any reason.

Step 3. After you have washed your hands, place the tape on the back of your hand and then pull it off one or two times. This removes some of the adhesive. The tape increases its stickiness while you are wearing it due to the moisture of the mouth.

Step 4. Place the tape in the position you want to use. There are four ways you can apply the tape:

- Place a small strip vertically from under your nose to just below your bottom lip.

- Place a slightly larger strip diagonally from one corner of your mouth to the other.

- Place two strips diagonally across your mouth (an *X*) from one corner to the other. For the first three, there is still an opening for you to mouth-breathe if necessary.

- Place one long strip from one corner of your mouth to the other so that it covers the lips completely and there is no way to open your mouth at all. This is the way I tape my lips. For this option especially, don't forget to create a tab by sticking one end of the tape onto itself.

Step 5. When taking the tape off in the morning, do it slowly and be extremely gentle and careful. There is the danger of tearing the skin on your lips if you remove the tape too quickly. Two other ways to remove the tape besides the tab are to (1) use your tongue to push the tape away from your lips slowly, or (2) wash your face and allow the water to soften the tape and make it easier to remove.

When I came back to the U.S. from Buteyko training in New Zealand, I was determined to become a nose breather. But each time I sat down in front of the computer, I found that I opened my mouth while typing. I broke the habit by taping my mouth every time I sat down at the computer until I learned to keep it shut.

I was taught that taping your mouth each night before bed for six months is ideal. After that, many people become nose breathers. That was also my experience. Even after 20 years, though, I still tape my mouth at night. For me it's like turning off the lights. Having a dry mouth in the morning is so uncomfortable, and mouth taping is so easy—why not? If the idea of mouth taping disturbs the romance of being in bed with your partner, you can always do it after the lights go out. The popularity and need to nasal-breathe while sleeping has opened a market for many kinds of mouth tape, which you can find on the Internet. Still, some people find tape just too uncomfortable and prefer to use a chin strap.

What about taping children's mouths? You'll have to decide and experiment for yourself depending on the age of your child. If you are uncomfortable with taping your child's mouth, check on them while they are sleeping and gently close their mouth with your fingers. Breaking the habit during the day may eventually teach them to keep their mouth closed while sleeping. You can make this a game by miming closing your mouth with your finger when you see them mouth-breathing.

Monitoring the Bedroom Atmosphere

It's important to keep a window open at night unless you're in an area where there is wildfire smoke. Make sure that the bedroom door stays open to circulate the air through the rest of the house. Doing so reduces the buildup of carbon-dioxide levels in the room. One or two people sleeping in a room with the windows closed can raise the room's atmosphere of carbon dioxide significantly. Average global atmosphere air levels of carbon dioxide in 2020 were 412.5 parts per million.[18] Sleeping in a bedroom without ventilation can raise CO_2 levels to 2,500 parts per million, causing headaches, fatigue, sleepiness, and difficulty thinking clearly during the day. Any increase in carbon dioxide above the outside atmospheric levels can start to impair brain functioning, especially when they reach 1,000 parts per million. Sitting in your living room without ventilation and watching TV or reading can also increase CO_2 levels.[19]

This situation is common in office buildings and classrooms that are not well ventilated. If you're thinking that keeping the windows closed and running an air purifier will help, please think again. Air purifiers do not scrub carbon dioxide. This was the one of the problems with the *Apollo 13* mission. Their carbon-dioxide scrubbers were failing, and if they hadn't fixed them, the astronauts would have suffocated due to the increase in CO_2. Driving in a car for long distances with the windows closed can raise CO_2 levels to 4,000 parts per million. How quickly that happens depends on how many people are in the car.

It is hard to know what the carbon-dioxide levels are anywhere in your house, office, or car or in other commonly used rooms without a monitor that registers CO_2. There are many air monitors on the market today, and if you decide to get one, make sure it registers CO_2 levels. I have two monitors, one for air quality that includes CO_2 levels and another that measures volatile organic compounds, which are harmful gases from household and work products, some of which cause cancer.

It is important for me, as a breathing educator working with people with many breathing challenges, to know and recommend these tools to help monitor the atmospheres you put yourself in. This includes restaurants, movie theaters, conference rooms, and workplaces. It is easy when you have breathing challenges to think something is wrong with you, when many times it is the air you are breathing. I carry a portable monitor to take into these places to know what the atmosphere is like and to let the owners and managers know that the environment is polluted and contributes to difficulty breathing among people with sensitive airways.

Optimizing Your Sleep Environment and Routine

1. Having a bedroom that is designed for sleep:[20]

    - Low light in preparation for sleep
    - Complete darkness while sleeping, including those little lights on devices
    - No electronic devices in the bedroom, including phones and computers

- If you are allergy prone:

    - Take out carpeting or at least clean it on a regular basis

    - Use hypoallergenic bedding

2. A change of your pillows on a regular basis to reduce the likelihood of mites

3. A regular bedtime schedule so that you go to sleep within the same hour each night

4. No alcohol within two hours of your bedtime; for some people, metabolizing alcohol can take up to 8 to 10 hours, depending on liver function

5. Limited caffeine intake, especially after early afternoon; for most people, the effects of caffeine last about 8 hours; for those more sensitive to caffeine, it can take even longer

6. Limit screen time before bed and/or wear blue-blocking glasses at night to lessen the activation of blue light, which can lower production of melatonin, a hormone that induces drowsiness. Many options and price ranges for blue-blocking glasses are available on the Internet and in stores

7. Before bed, do a practice that helps ease the tensions of the day, such as meditation

8. A cool bedroom—67 degrees F (18 degrees C) is optimal

Increasing the Flow of Breath

Find a sleep specialist if you have signs of breathing-disordered sleep.[21] Providers who specialize in Buteyko Breathing Education; sleep dentistry; ear, nose, and throat doctors; and sleep specialists offer a number of options to increase the flow of breath, which may be limited by inflammation within the airways or structural constraints:

- Breathing education
- Orofacial myofunctional therapy (OMT)
- A continuous positive airway pressure (CPAP) machine to regulate and increase the force of air
- Dental procedures to widen and reshape the upper palate to create more room for the tongue to rest comfortably
- Laser therapy to reduce inflammation in the throat and tongue
- A mouth guard to help keep the lower jaw in place
- Surgery

My wife, Nell, who until recently was able to sleep quietly most nights, began to have episodes of loud snoring and difficulty exhaling, which created pressure in her chest. Then as she'd drop into deep sleep, her respiration became quiet. With less volume of air circulating, her airways began to collapse. She stopped getting enough oxygen, her body struggled to breathe, and she woke up, her autonomic nervous system on high alert because of the lack of oxygen.

As James Nestor writes in *Breath*, humans today have smaller mouths with less room for breathing than our ancestors did. So Nell and I went to see a dentist who specializes in dental sleep medicine and breathing-disordered sleep, and that turned out to be the case with her. The airway behind her tongue had become narrow, and when she relaxed, her tongue and soft palate fell back into her throat, leaving little room for breathing.

After conferring with a colleague in the Buteyko work and an orofacial myofunctional therapist, she decided to try tongue therapy and a mouth guard as first steps, and then reevaluate. The therapist recommending doing the orofacial myofunctional therapy first so that any further solutions would be more effective if this aspect of breathing health was in place. Nell also went to see an ear, nose, and throat doctor since her turbinates were inflamed. Changing her diet to anti-inflammatory foods, along with some saline spray, solved this problem, keeping her airway clean and lubricated. There are many solutions, and we need to find what works best for us.

I was consulting with a longtime friend about his sleep. One day his therapist on Zoom said to him, "You look terrible. Are you getting enough sleep?" He knew that he was having trouble sleeping, waking up two hours after falling asleep, often in an activated state, taking a couple of hours to go to sleep again. I suggested that he get a sleep study (polysomnography), a comprehensive test for diagnosing sleep disorders that records your brain waves, the oxygen level in your blood, your heart rate, and your breathing, as well as eye and leg movements during sleep.

It came back that he has sleep apnea, and the recommendation was to use a CPAP machine, which he found difficult, although he was feeling better. I suggested he next see a sleep dentist to evaluate his facial and tongue structures, and perhaps also see an orofacial myofunctional therapist. He saw both and is currently wearing a dental device to keep his jaw from falling backward into his airway. It turned out he has restrictions of the movement of his tongue. He is tongue-tied and is having those ties released so that he can place his tongue in the proper position for breathing, swallowing, and sleeping. He is also inquiring, with his therapist, into some psychological patterns that disturb his sleep—ongoing anxiety from the belief that he always has to be on the go, accomplishing something all the time, which makes it difficult for his system to relax.

The combination of the myofunctional therapy, releasing his tongue ties, the dental device, learning to nasal breathe, slowing and relaxing his breathing, and psychotherapy has helped him get better sleep and reduce the incidences of apnea. He told me he had no idea how important sleep was to his overall sense of well-being and health. He is much happier now and pleased to have learned so much about the importance of sleep.

EXPLORATION

Falling Asleep and Staying Asleep

As you prepare for sleep, notice the movement of air as it enters and leaves your nostrils. This can have a relaxing effect and slow your breathing.

Then ask yourself, *What is the quality of my breathing and my body's energy? Is it soothing? Relaxing? Energized? Scattered?* What sensations do you notice? How and where is your body resting on the support beneath you? If your energy is running quick, you may need to spend some time quieting yourself before trying to fall asleep.

Here are five exercises that can help you prepare for sleep. You can also practice these if you wake up during the night.

1. Mini-Pause—see Appendix D, "Buteyko Breathing Education Exercises."

2. Nose Clearing—see Appendix D, "Buteyko Breathing Education Exercises."

3. Reducing Hidden Hyperventilation—see page 163.

4. Being Breathed: *Sa~Ha*—see Appendix G, "Further Explorations."

5. Humming—studies show that humming for 20 minutes before bed is effective in reducing stuffiness during sleep.[22]

REDUCING HIDDEN HYPERVENTILATION

You can do this exploration at your own pace, in any position. If you wake up during the night, you can do it lying right where you are.

To practice this exercise, breathe in and out through your nose at whatever rate and depth you are currently breathing. There is no manipulating your breath to fit a certain rate or depth. The same is true when the instruction says "pause." However long you can pause in that moment is fine. Note that it says "pause for the count of." The count is in your mind. There is no special duration to pause each time. It may take you only one second or less to pause for the count of two. Or it might take you three or four seconds. It is the same for how long you pause each time as you go up the scale to six. As you count down from pausing for the count of six, you can expect that the breathing rate will slow down and the pausing for the counts will take longer.

Physiologically, the pausing is increasing the baseline of carbon dioxide, which is facilitating the release of oxygen from the blood to the cells and helping you enter a state of feeling rested and settled, which is what you want to help you fall asleep.

I repeat this exercise when needed, and I find it always to be a good reminder. Using *Sa~Ha* while doing this can make it even more effective.

- Breathe in and out through your nose twice. Pause for the count of two at the end of the second exhale. Repeat.

- Breathe in and out through your nose twice. Pause for the count of three at the end of the second exhale. Repeat.

- Breathe in and out through your nose twice. Pause for the count of four at the end of the second exhale. Repeat.

- Breathe in and out through your nose twice. Pause for the count of five at the end of the second exhale. Repeat.

- Breathe in and out through your nose twice. Pause for the count of six at the end of the second exhale. Repeat.

- Breathe in and out through your nose twice. Pause for the count of five at the end of the second exhale. Repeat.

- Breathe in and out through your nose twice. Pause for the count of four at the end of the second exhale. Repeat.

- Breathe in and out through your nose twice. Pause for the count of three at the end of the second exhale. Repeat.

- Breathe in and out through your nose twice. Pause for the count of two at the end of the second exhale. Repeat.

You can repeat this exercise as often as needed until you fall back to sleep.

If counting to six feels too challenging, stop at a lower number and go backward from there. If you still can't get back to sleep, get out of bed and do this exercise until you get tired.

Some people wake up during the night in fight-or-flight mode. When the body is not getting enough oxygen as a result of breathing-disordered sleep, it triggers this response. Other times you may be having thoughts you can't shut off. The release of adrenaline will speed up your heart rate and breathing, inducing a feeling of restlessness, activation, anxiety, or panic. As I mentioned earlier, the adrenaline can take a while to clear before the body can settle down.

Sometimes trying to slow your breathing, as in the exercises outlined here, won't work because movement is what is needed. Getting out of bed and moving around can help, until you feel yourself settling back down. Then the breathing exercises can help get you back to sleep.

PART IV

TRANSFORMING YOUR WORLD

AND

YOUR LIFE, ONE BREATH AT A TIME

As you breathe in, cherish yourself.
As you breathe out, cherish all beings.

— THE DALAI LAMA

CHAPTER SIXTEEN

BREATHING WITH PAIN

All healing originally resides in the human breathing system.

— RUDOLF STEINER, AUTHOR, ARCHITECT, AND
THE FOUNDER OF ANTHROPOSOPHY

Pain can take your breath away. A moment of physical or emotional suffering can be so intense that you gasp and find it difficult to breathe. Adrenaline and cortisol course through your body, and you're caught in the terror of what the body and mind are actually going through and fearful that the pain may never go away. Someone supporting you might suggest, "Just breathe," or "Take a deep breath." Both are good advice.

I prefer to invite someone to "take a breath from deep within." And, of course, to use their nose as they try to find equilibrium. When instructed to take a "deep breath," most people open their mouth to breathe in and out and lift their shoulders to suck in more air. Trying to breathe from "deep within" encourages you to breathe with your belly and diaphragm, increasing your lung capacity and getting the satisfying breath you need at that moment to signal your nervous system that you're trying to settle down. Taking a "deep breath" while breathing in and out through your mouth can keep you using your chest to breathe, making it more difficult to get a satisfying breath and continuing to support the chemistry of danger.

After finishing a painful race in the 2022 Winter Olympics, the South Korean women's speed-skating team needed to restore their breathing. Each of the four women bent over and, with their mouths closed, used their bellies to breathe. There was no gasping. I find it important after exercising to take the time to restore breathing to its resting rhythm. Otherwise you might continue to breathe as if you were still exercising.

Pain is an abstract term to describe an aggregate of sensations. If you use words like *tight, stinging, sore, tearing, sharp, hot,* and *piercing,* you can address the specific pain you're feeling. Your health-care support team is more likely to be able to help if you describe specific sensations. *Pain* is shorthand, an abstract concept that makes it harder to get at the actual situation and easy for fear levels to rise as you lose the impulse to contact the specific sensations. When you examine any sensations closely, you discover the ever-changing nature of pain, allowing you to enter into a living process with it.

Let's say you feel pain in your back. It is sharp or dull? Does it feel searing? Are you having spasms? Stiffness? Achiness? Tenderness? Tingling? Weakness? Numbness? What part of your back? Do you feel hot or cold or somewhere in between? Crunchy? Compacted? Grabbing? Tight? When identifying these *sensations*, you are in direct conversation with the complex of pain.

Try it. Pick a place that feels uncomfortable and say, "I have a pain here." Does that help you or others address the issue? Then ask yourself, *What am I sensing? What sensations do I feel?* Name that sensation and say, "This place of pain feels hot," or "This place of pain feels tight." Listen to how that sounds and whether it gives you more information about your pain.

It can be hard to understand another person's pain and easier to empathize with a specific sensation. It's more direct, and we may have had the same sensation at one time or another. If we are more direct, solutions may reveal themselves.

Once you're able to identify your actual sensations, you can *breathe with* them and learn from them. You may recall that at the end of Chapter 3, "The Sensuous Nature of Breathing," there's an exploration called "Breathing with Sensations." That practice can be useful when working with pain. Practicing it when you're not in pain will give you the skills when needed.

As you breathe *with* the sensations of the pain, at first it might become more intense. After a while the intensity may dissipate as you continue to bring the awareness of your breathing to the area of pain. What previously felt stuck may now be in movement, and your perception of pain changes too. As you stay present, there may be more in the background that you hadn't noticed.

Pain isolates. It draws us away from direct experience. We simply wish it wasn't there. We want to ignore it, but if we do, it may become intolerable. The pain gets louder, we want it to go away even more, and our sense of fragmentation increases: *This pain keeps me from feeling whole within myself.* Our psyches as well as our biology desire to be coherent and whole.

Breathing with, consciously providing the life force of breath to what has been isolated, invites the area of isolation to rejoin the rest of the body. You never know beforehand how your body will respond. It is a living *process,* always attempting to fulfill its biological imperative to reach for what serves the health of the organism. While you may have a certain desired outcome, keep that in the background as you meet, in open attention, whatever you encounter. What will be most beneficial is simply noticing whatever you become aware of.

Pain usually includes contraction and impermeability. Nutrient supply, including blood flow, slows, and the removal of waste products stagnates as tightened muscles decrease movement. Our tissues are trying to limit movements that might cause more pain. If our discomfort is in a limb and we try to move to test our level of pain—such as flexion, extension, abduction, and adduction or rotations, up and down, side to side, and around—it may cause more pain and more contraction, a recoil. The lack of movement can become wired into the nervous system until we lose our range of motion, maybe even after the pain has dissipated. Allowing the *wave* of our breath to stimulate nonlinear movement can remind the tissue of other possibilities. The gentle movement of breath invites what has been painfully isolated back into the whole of the body, even if just for a moment to begin with.

A few days before Emilie Conrad left her body, I stood at the foot of her bed as she lifted her head ever so slightly to look at me and said, "Robert, *the kernel of attention is really small.*" I knew this would be the last teaching I'd receive from her, and that lesson has stayed with me ever since and informed how I attend to sensations when they arise, even painful ones.

When a complex of sensations is inviting my attention, I ask myself, *And what's underneath that?* using the kernel of attention to go more deeply into the tissue layers where the sensations live and deepen the inquiry. I ask the same question over and over while *breathing with* whatever is revealed into my awareness, until I know I can't go any deeper. I have gone through the eye of the needle, and the complex of sensation often brings me to a new perception of myself and my pain that is both surprising and, at the same time, familiar. This kind of intention, attention, and inquiry takes time and practice.

Over the years, some of my pains have revealed emotional memories, mostly from childhood, which were obscured. After inquiring for a while and repeatedly marrying my awareness, my breathing, and the movement of my breathable body with the site of the pain, I would notice that the pain was no longer present. I wasn't trying to make it disappear. I suppose the pain signals had served their purpose. Then, later, another complex of pain would arise, more limiting than the previous one, and I would receive it as an invitation to do more inquiry and work with it the same way. This living process has been with me for many years, always taking me deeper into my body, deeper into my sense of being okay and whole, revealing more of what was hidden and protected that was at the same time longing to be seen and to rejoin the whole.

This intuitive trajectory has brought me back from the despair and isolation of my childhood.

Not all pain can be "worked" this way. Some requires a different kind of intervention. If you break your arm, you need to see a doctor.

EXPLORATION

BREATHING WITH PAIN

I'll tell you right now, the doors to the world
of the wild Self are few but precious.
If you have a deep scar, that is a door, if you have
an old, old story, that is a door.

— CLARISSA PINKOLA ESTÉS, *WOMEN WHO*
RUN WITH THE WOLVES

Place yourself in a comfortable position that supports breathing. Then take a baseline: *What and where is the discomfort or pain I want to focus on? What is the pain level now?*

Turn your attention to the area where you feel the sensations of pain. You don't have to name or be specific about it; only be aware that you are focusing on some particular sensation. You can also place your hands on the location and use the sound of "hum," *O,* or *E* for more internal awareness. You will know you are there when you stop calling it "pain" and are curious about what you are *feeling.*

On the next inhale, *breathe with* what you are experiencing (noticing), and continue to blend your awareness with the movement of your breath and with that sensation as you exhale. Then on the next cycle or two of breathing, take a moment to notice where you felt that sensation while you were *breathing with* it and inquire if it feels the same or has changed somehow. Has there been movement within the complex of the pain? If there has, then ask, *And what is beneath that?* or *What else is there to notice?*

If it has not changed, *breathe with* it again and ask yourself the same questions. Repeat until you feel that you need rest or that you've gone as deeply as you can for now. Go into open attention, simply noticing what arrives in your awareness and what that means for you. This is the beginning of meeting the sensations of pain on their own terms.

When you focus awareness and *breathe with* the sensations of pain, you may be drawn to another sensation in that area or somewhere else in your body. Follow that for a while. What is painful in one area might be connected to something or somewhere else. By connecting the dots, you may be entering the "complex dynamic" of the pain syndrome, realizing the connections that need to be experienced. This is a multilayered approach to working with the map of the body through sensations. It may take many times exploring multiple layers of inner connections before one day you realize the pain is no longer there or your relationship with it has changed.

As you develop a sense of movement in a previously "stuck" area, try to keep these movements and areas in your awareness as you go through your everyday activities. When you do so, the difficult areas can be integrated back into the body's full range of motion, providing healing through the medicine of movement. The contractions that have reduced the capacity of the tissues to receive the nourishment of breath may now be more receptive and permeable.

CHAPTER SEVENTEEN

BREATHING
WITH ANXIETY

If you want to conquer the anxiety of life,
live in the moment, live in the breath.

— AMIT RAY, *OM CHANTING AND MEDITATION*[1]

Hundreds of millions of years ago, the first defense against a life-threatening situation was to freeze and play dead. As time moved forward, two other options developed—to run away or fight back. These responses to threats are still part of our autonomic nervous system. They are also our responses to stress, and they're often automatic, not a choice. We freeze when our fear is too overwhelming for us to move, and we run or fight if our reflexes sense that doing so would be the best option.

Just 300,000 years ago, brain size in early *Homo sapiens* entered the range of present-day humans,[2] and we developed a large prefrontal cortex and, with it, a wild imagination. Today we can sit down for morning coffee and read about wars, public health catastrophes, wealth inequality, and global climate change on our smartphones. Although our cerebral cortex can distinguish what's happening in the present moment from nonproximate dangers, our ancient defense strategies—fight-flight-freeze—arise instantly, including anxious breathing and the impulse to act immediately. Our nervous systems often don't know the difference.

The key to reining in these primal impulses is *presence*. When we become present with what our five senses are perceiving, imaginal or nonproximate fears can fade into the background, allowing for an appropriate response. And nothing is more immediately available for us to focus on than our breathing and the body's movement in response to breath. Yes, climate change and mass extinctions are real and extreme threats, but our system cannot sustain a 24-7 fight-flight-freeze response.

After years of meeting with people in fight-or-flight mode who are not actually threatened in real time, I believe the option of "being present," widely discussed in the developing mindfulness movement, based on ancient Buddhist teachings, may be an attempt to evolve an alternative way of responding—to dangers that reside in our thoughts and imaginations. Futurist Barbara Marx Hubbard described it this way:

> Our media, which are like a planetary nervous system, are far more sensitive to breakdowns than to breakthroughs. They filter out our creativity and successes, considering them less newsworthy than violence, war, and dissent. When we read newspapers and watch television news, we feel closer to a death in the social body than to an awakening. Yes, something is dying; however, the media do not recognize that *something is also being born*.[3]

What's being born is a rewiring that allows us to be *present* with our physical reality in this moment. Asking ourselves what we are smelling, tasting, seeing, hearing, and touching is what is most immediate.

For me, as a breathing educator, my most immediate access to a sensing body is to tune in to the movement and inner touch of breath. Other ways I step away from the fears that drive the sympathetic nervous system and deplete vitality are to connect with nature, beauty, and other people. Connection is a basic human need that can help us reconnect with resting and settling.

The term *stress* as it is currently used was adopted by endocrinologist Hans Selye in 1936. He also coined the term *eustress* ("good stress") to describe a moderate psychological stress that may be beneficial for us in the way that "good pain" can help build muscle. But when we're exposed to constant distress, the body's systems—including the immune, digestive, circulatory, nervous systems—and organ functions begin to break down. Selye called this general adaptation syndrome (GAS), and we can see it throughout society today with the prevalence of heart disease, digestive disorders, asthma, breathing-disordered sleep, and generalized anxiety. Manufacturing and dispensing medications to suppress these symptoms constitutes a multibillion-dollar industry.[4]

A common folk remedy for calming anxiety is to inhale as much air as you can and then let it all out through your mouth, and repeat. This instruction is usually given after a period of tension, overstimulation, emotional upset, unexplainable rapid breathing, or shallow breathing (using your chest, not your diaphragm). If performed repeatedly, it can lead to hyperventilation and a tightening of the breathing muscles and can limit the capacity of the lungs to open and fill. That, in turn, can make you feel like you cannot get a deep breath or you need one, a condition that can become chronic and debilitating.

Taking a deep breath might help you feel relaxed for a moment, but your old breathing habits and behaviors will return, and before you know it, you'll need another deep breath. First, you can't let out all the air in your lungs or they'd collapse. Some air is always retained. And mouth-breathing reduces the flow of oxygen to the cells by lowering the levels of CO_2 (the Bohr effect), compromising the cells' ability to provide the energy needed to power the body's systems.

The need for more air is real, but rather than taking big breaths through your mouth, try *slowing down*, breathing with your nose, and returning your awareness to the internal movements of breathing. Using the signals of anxiety as a request by your nervous system to bring your attention back to the sensation of breathing can help you slow down and self-regulate. Other ways to relieve the stress of oxygen deprivation are (1) making sure you're in a posture that eases the flow of breathing rather than restricts it, (2) feeling the support of what is beneath you on each exhale, and (3) practicing *Sa~Ha* breathing.

When I'm anxious, I feel it in my chest. Sometimes the onset is quick, and I'm cold throughout my body, especially in my hands and feet, shivering and feeling tight and compressed. My eyes get superfocused on what I'm looking at, scanning for the threat. I don't hear birds singing or see clouds in the sky. While this is happening, my mouth usually drops open, my tongue is somewhere in the middle of my mouth, and I'm breathing quickly and shallowly, using only my chest. My breath stays caught in this small space, and I can't get enough air to ease or nourish me. My belly and diaphragm aren't moving.

My mind turns to thoughts of survival: *How am I going to make it through this? What can I do to make it better?* I feel so awful inside that I'm screaming to get out of my body—to find solutions outside of my inner experience. Even if these solutions were available, I'm too anxious to make any of these changes. Over years of observing this, I've learned to use my breathing behavior to move from anxiety to rest and, on my better days, to peace of body and mind. I try to introduce slow, quiet breathing, making sure that my tongue, lips, and teeth are in the correct positions; my eyes are utilizing peripheral vision; and I have a strong sense of support beneath me.

When we're anxious, we generally breathe shallowly, high up in the chest with a speedy rhythm. When we're depressed, our breath is small and shallow, proceeding at a slow rate. Neither extreme supports long-term health. If we're anxious much of the time, we may be pushing down fear, anger, or grief, leaving us suppressed and depressed. All behaviors express themselves within the body's dynamic and our breathing patterns. It's important to learn to rest and settle, to move away from being anxious about what is happening in the moment, worrying about the future, or perseverating about the past.

To *rest* is to cease work or movement in order to relax, refresh, and recover strength. Relaxation is a movement of allowing. When was the last time you really relaxed, without tension, with thoughts that were peaceful? For many, the answer is "Not for a long time." How many times a day do you *allow* the ease and pleasure of an experience?

To *settle* is to resolve a conflict. We need ways to rest and settle, to remove the tension from our body so we can feel refreshed and ready to take on each next moment of life. We can practice yoga, Pilates, Continuum, or meditation; or enjoy a massage, exercise, watch TV, read, take a walk, or share time with a friend. Most important is to have a *supportive atmosphere* that pleases you aesthetically and spiritually, since primarily you're building a connection with yourself.

Recall a time you felt deeply settled. Take a moment and check in with how that feels in your body—the movement of your breathing and how your body was "being breathed" by the flow of air in and out. Feel the physical reality of your body in relation to what's beneath you, and notice the support you are receiving from the earth. Deep relaxation and feeling supported can serve as touchstones for what resting and breathing slowly are like.

Resonance frequency breathing (RFB) is a slow, relaxed diaphragmatic breathing at around three to seven breaths per minute that has a regulating effect on the autonomic nervous system and the circulatory system. When practiced in the right conditions, it calms the body's fight-or-flight response and increases the activity of the parasympathetic nervous system and the vagus nerve, which are important in helping us cope with stress and facilitating healing. When we breathe at our resonance frequency, our respiratory, cardiovascular, and autonomic nervous systems synchronize and work together.

Some people practice RFB for 5.5 seconds in and 5.5 seconds out, 11 seconds per breath. I prefer 4 seconds in and 6 seconds out. There are apps and programs that can guide you in this rhythm. (See the Online Resources listed in the back of the book, and especially the website of Rosalba Courtney.)[5]

EXPLORATION

Calming Anxiety in 81 Seconds

One of the things that scares people during an anxiety attack is that the heart rate speeds up and feels like a drum in the chest. This Buteyko exercise can take around 81 seconds to stop an anxiety or panic attack. I have used it many times with clients with great success. This exercise differs from the one I suggested when you wake up in the middle of the night or are trying to fall asleep. This one is actually timed. You can do it for yourself, or you can help someone in need of stopping an anxiety or panic attack.

These are some things you can do when you notice that you're feeling anxious:

1. Close your mouth and breathe through your nose.

2. Place your tongue at the roof of your mouth with your lips lightly touching and teeth a couple of millimeters apart.

3. Find ground to support your body. If you're walking, feel your feet meeting the earth. If you're sitting, put yourself in the horse-rider position and find support for your sit bones and your feet. If you're lying down, scan to find where you feel supported.

4. Put your hands on your heart and belly, and breathe with an awareness of the connection your hands are making; the texture of the tissues beneath them; and how those places are moving with each breath, comforting your heart, your diaphragm, and the part of your nervous system that lives in the belly—your gut brain and the feelings there.

5. Repeat these steps as often as needed; then proceed with counting your breath. The timing is in seconds. You can use a stopwatch, a wristwatch, a clock, your phone, or

any timepiece. Each time you say that is one second. The count only goes up to six seconds. You must reverse the count when you get to six seconds and come back down to two seconds. Here's the sequence:

- Breathe in for two seconds and out for three seconds.
- Pause for two seconds.
- Breathe in for two seconds and out for three seconds.
- Pause for three seconds.
- Breathe in for two seconds and out for three seconds.
- Pause for four seconds.
- Breathe in for two seconds and out for three seconds.
- Pause for five seconds.
- Breathe in for two seconds and out for three seconds.
- Pause for six seconds.
- Breathe in for two seconds and out for three seconds.
- Pause for five seconds.
- Breathe in for two seconds and out for three seconds.
- Pause for four seconds.
- Breathe in for two seconds and out for three seconds.
- Pause for three seconds.
- Breathe in for two seconds and out for three seconds.
- Pause for two seconds.

6. Finish, and repeat if necessary. Take a walk in nature and use your five senses to attune to your surroundings. If you can't go outside, check in with each of your senses one at a time. What are you hearing? Smelling? Tasting? Touching? Seeing?

The sensations we call *anxiety* are vibrations moving quickly, accompanied by a breathing pattern that is quick almost to the point of breathlessness. You can feel these vibrations in the chest (rapid breathing) or in the belly (queasiness). When they're in your chest, you're breathing shallowly, unable to get enough air—a pattern that, unless you're exercising vigorously, is out of sync with your body. When the body is in a state of fight-or-flight or highly activated, it releases the hormone adrenaline, the body's defense against fear (essentially, the body's "speed"). Once adrenaline has been released, it can be difficult to slow your breathing down.

In addition to facilitating a quick escape from danger, adrenaline has these effects on the body:

- Decreases our ability to feel pain

- Temporarily increases strength

- Sharpens focus, which allows us to think quickly and form a clear plan to escape

- Increases the heart rate (which can feel like the heart racing)

- Redirects blood toward the muscles, causing a surge in energy or shaking limbs

- Relaxes the airways to give the muscles more oxygen, which may cause breathing to become shallow

- Dilates the pupils to let more light enter the eyes

- Induces sweating as a reaction to stress

- Causes light-headedness due to changes in blood and oxygen supply

- Changes our body temperature as a result of the blood redirection[6]

The body breaks down adrenaline through a chemical process, which vigorous movement and vigorous breathing can help. This is why it may be difficult to slow your breathing while your body is asking for activity. This often happens with sleep apnea, when the body is oxygen depleted for a long enough time to cause the nervous system to go on alert and wake you up gasping for air. An adrenaline rush can last a while, as I've said before.

When there is a more generalized state of anxiety, the frequency or vibration (the speed and pace of the movement) of the energy of anxiety varies depending on the area of the body where you're feeling it. Anxiety in the chest might have a different frequency than anxiety in the belly. They feel different, but both point to nervousness, worry, concern, unease, apprehension, disquiet, fretfulness, angst, fear, or any of the other names given to this experience.

Generalized anxiety is not only about clear-and-present dangers; it can also be connected to unmetabolized past trauma stored in the body—buzzing in your head, pain in a shoulder, tension in your hands . . . anywhere. With exploration, you may experience these places vibrating. We may need to step outside the reactive frequency to gain insight into whether the trigger was something new or a habitual response to protect you against retraumatization.

Tensional *patterns* that indicate anxiety, like moving frantically, shaking, or feeling scattered, can arise even when there isn't an obvious trigger. These ongoing muscular patterns can dictate the tempo of our breathing and its capacity to nourish. And the patterns keep asserting themselves. Becoming conscious of them can be the beginning of a shift.

If you breathe consciously while maintaining awareness of the exact location of the anxious vibration and its frequency, you can slow your breathing and move from being reactive to being responsive when you see that it's simply a habitual pattern. If you practice awareness of sensations and slowed-down breathing when anxiety isn't present or when it's mild, you'll have more skill to do so when it appears strongly. When I have this experience, I allow my body to "breathe" me using the *Sa~Ha* meditation practice, which opens up more space in my lungs and body. As the space opens, the frequency of breathing shifts to one that relaxes and nourishes.

Imagine a small box with 10 marbles inside it. When you shake the box, the marbles have a particular sound. Now put the same

10 marbles into a bigger box and shake them again. The sound will be different. The marbles are moving at a different frequency because the space is bigger, and it takes longer before they hit the sides of the box. The same is true for the vibrations of anxiety within the body. Enlarge the size of the container (the lungs and the body), and you will transition to a calmer frequency.

Your autonomic nervous system's responses to trauma and worry are probably well-grooved patterns. If it's a freeze response, you shut down, either holding yourself still or collapsing your head over your rib basket to make your breathing small so it won't be detected. Playing dead is hard work, and the fear stays buried deep in the body. When you're having a fight-or-flight response, you become hypervigilant.

Our *kinesphere* is the space surrounding our body—in movement or in stillness, in all directions and at all levels. It is close to the body and as far as we can reach with our arms and legs, and we perceive this "personal space" through our senses. We can physically and intuitively be aware of what's in front and in back of us, on either side, above, and below. If we've been hurt in any area of the body, we can lose the ability to perceive our "personal space" around that spot. Unable to perceive what might be around us in that area, we can't feel completely safe. Not knowing creates anxiety.

I learned about kinesphere from movement and Rolfing teacher Hubert Godard. He described a young man with scoliosis, an unnatural curvature of the spine, who came to him for body-work. His father was violent, and every time the young man did something his father didn't like, he would reach out and smack him. The son learned to curve his spine to stay out of his father's reach, while at the same time reducing his ability to track his personal space on that side of his body.

I came to one of Hubert's workshops with a sprained ankle, a common occurrence for me. He said the problem wasn't with my ankle but my left eye. I wasn't using that eye to see what was in my personal space, causing me to lose sight of where I walked—a loss of *proprioception*, knowing where I was in space. I walked back and forth in the room so other participants could see a baseline of how I walked. He then did some bodywork on my eye and told me to walk again. I was much more grounded and using my eye more effectively.

Nell was in the room, and when I looked at her, I started to cry and asked her, "If I change, will you still love me?" I had been so protected until then, and suddenly I felt raw and vulnerable. A few minutes later I had a memory of my mother being so drunk at the dinner table that her face would fall into her food, triggering my father's rage. I couldn't stand the sight of her, and I turned my left eye "off."

Later Nell commented that she always felt more comfortable walking on my right side—that she didn't feel seen when on my left. Over time, I practiced using my left eye to see what was around me, and I discovered that it was more than my eye. The whole left side of my body and particularly my shoulder held this fear and disgust over losing my mother to drink. Vibrations of fear were buried deep in my shoulder, ribs, and lungs, limiting my capacity to breathe fully.

There are other nervous systems in our body as well: The walls of our stomach and our entire alimentary canal are lined with a network of neurons named the *enteric nervous system*, also called our *second brain* or *gut brain*. The alimentary canal, approximately 29 feet long, is the pathway of digestion from the mouth to the anus, and it has more nerve endings in it than our spinal cord. The gut brain influences our moods, breathing, and sense of well-being. It reports to our brain by sending messages to the cerebral cortex via the vagus nerve.[7]

Sometimes when you're out in nature or with someone you trust, your belly might relax and you feel safe. At other times, you might feel "sick to your stomach," activated by a feeling of disgust. These responses, many of which don't register consciously, provide a lot of information. When something feels "off," you might sense it through discomfort in your belly. A tight belly inhibits the movement of the diaphragm, a primary respiratory muscle tucked up right beneath the stomach, and when your belly is tight, your breathing might be shallow. Sometimes, to allow the belly to soften so you can breathe with ease, you might have to bring undigested recent (as well as long-past) emotional events into awareness. It's always important to go slowly when you're exploring your belly.

If we've been holding our belly, sometimes when we finally relax—during a massage or while meditating or doing a releasing movement—our digestive system might announce that it's coming back online by gurgling. I highly recommend Allison Post and Stephen Cavaliere's book *Unwinding the Belly*, which offers ways to touch your belly that help release tension. Practicing some of these has been a great comfort and helped me realize how much anxiety I've stored in my belly.

EXPLORATION

BREATHING WITH YOUR BELLY

For many people, the belly is a vulnerable place. If this exploration seems to go too fast or even be invasive, please see the longer, gentler exploration in Appendix G, "Befriending Your Belly."

Begin this exploration by lying on your back with your knees bent and feet flat on the floor (or you can place a bolster or a pillow under your knees). This allows the diaphragm to be free to move without the constriction of the belly organs. It's okay to have a small pillow under your neck.

When you feel ready, bring both hands to your belly and tune in to the relationship between your hands and your breathing belly as you breathe in and out. What do you notice?

I've practiced this exploration for many years and continue to do so at least once a day, resting and gently rubbing my hands on my belly as I breathe. I find it soothing and informative. I listen for gurgling, which tells me I'm softening and resting. Sometimes I have one hand on my belly and the other on my heart.

As a child, I was overweight and wore "husky" clothes, and in college my nickname was Buddha Belly. It was all strange to me, because in my mind I saw myself as a lean, graceful dancer. My body and my body image were not in alignment, and I grew up ashamed of my belly.

This exploration led me to soften and release stored memories and shame. Without the protective big belly, anything in this area was terrifying. I realized I was afraid of my sensuous nature. I would often go on diets to reduce the size of my belly. As soon as I reached a weight that felt comfortable and sensuous, I would start to overeat again. This went on for too many years to count.

As my belly relaxed over the years and learned to be an essential part of my breathing, I've come to feel safe with myself, enjoying the pleasure of my breathing and my sensuous nature without the enlarged belly that holds so much fear. I no longer overeat.

I invite you into this world of your breathing belly. Trust your intuition as you develop an intimate relationship with your belly, touching it in ways that feel comforting and loving. Allow your belly to guide your breathing. There are many ways of breathing with anxiety, and they can all help. Be tender with yourself. Go slowly and mindfully.

CHAPTER EIGHTEEN

AWAKENING TO SILENCE

Our breath, like our heartbeat,
is the most reliable rhythm in our lives.
When we become attuned to this constant rhythm,
our breath can gradually teach us
to come back to the original silence of the mind.

— DONNA FARHI, YOGA TEACHER AND AUTHOR

In the mid-1990s, I attended a men's gathering at Bear Lake, California. There were around 50 men of various ages and professions gathered to meet, play, talk, and develop a sense of community—to help end the feeling of isolation among men.

On the first day, we met in small groups to get to know each other. Our group's leader invited us to think about a sound that felt appropriate to our nature, to write it on a piece of paper, and then when called upon, to make that sound out loud—a simple exercise to get us to use our voices and hear each other. I have no idea why, but I picked *silence* as my sound, and when my turn came, I said nothing; I just stayed silent and still. It took a while for the group to "get" what I was offering, and then I explained that to me silence is a sound and being silent felt like my most authentic response in that moment.

At birth, we take our first inhale. At death, we ride out on our last exhale. Each inhale throughout our lifetime is a recapitulation of that first breath, animating and igniting our life force. We are born again and again, made manifest in a moment of creation. As the inhale dissolves into the exhale, we gradually end the cycle, not knowing whether there will be another breath. At the end of the exhale, as the body rests awaiting the arrival of the inhale, the beating of our hearts—the desire for life—calls forth the next breath. Twenty thousand times a day we repeat this cycle of birth and death—body, mind, spirit, and heart, all contained and moving within the cycle of each breath.

When listening to a baby sleeping, we might wonder if they're breathing at all. Healthy babies' breathing is silent, and there's little movement to indicate that they're inhaling and exhaling. When breathing is relaxed and easy, it's noiseless; there's no sound coming from the movement of air in and out. When breathing is noisy, it's an indication that we're breathing *too much*, what Dr. Buteyko called *hidden hyperventilation*, trying to move too much air too quickly. Or there may be a structural problem in the airway that impedes the flow of air, thus creating sounds.

The openings of the nose allow only so much breath in and out at a time, and our lungs prefer that we breathe at a speed, volume, and temperature they can accommodate without stress. When breath is moving too quickly, the body constricts these openings to slow the pace and reduce the volume. We know intuitively that when someone is snoring loudly, they're having a hard time breathing. Silence indicates an easy flow of breath and a relaxed musculature throughout the body. With practice, you can learn to listen to and quiet your breathing.

I have tinnitus, which is a ringing or other noise in the ears. Many reasons have been suggested for tinnitus, including one hypothesis that some New Yorkers get it from listening to the high-pitched squeal of subway wheels pulling into a station. Tinnitus can also be the result of nerve damage—for example, from listening to high-decibel sounds at a very loud concert. My tinnitus is "brain noise," which I experience as a persistent static. Yet there are times my tinnitus completely stops.

When I was on the swimming team in high school, the moments I loved the most were being underwater in silence. When I'm out in nature or somewhere else deeply quiet, the world becomes more vivid and I feel restored. At those times, I can touch the silence behind all sound and experience a sense of calm. I breathe *with* the sound of silence and find that I am touching the calmness inherent in silence.

I doubt that my brain noise is based on nerve damage. If it were nerve damage, I don't think it would turn off at times. When I'm in a deep meditative state, it feels as if there's a shift in my brain energy. I'm no longer distracted by the tinnitus and more available to experience other sensations.

A decibel is the unit used to measure the intensity of a sound. In general parlance, the decibel level means the amount of loudness. The decibel level of people speaking is about 60. Leaves rustling is about 30 decibels. Anything below 30 is considered silent. In the *anechoic* (non-echoing) *chamber* at the Orfield Laboratories in Minnesota—a room designed to stop echoes—the decibel level is minus 9.4, a silence that can be described as "deafening" and disorienting. Places in the natural world that are quiet do have animal and other nonindustrial sounds to help us orient.

We orient—knowing where we are in space—through sound. We identify as human through our sound, which is different from other sounds we hear in nature or in civilization. When we listen deeply, we can hear the sound of silence that is *behind* all other sounds. It's not *complete* silence but a tolerable, even delicious, deep quiet—the field that holds all other sounds. The quieter the surrounding area, the more our ears can tune in to quieter sounds. When conditions are quiet, we can hear our heartbeat, the movement of air in our lungs, our digestion, and other biological functions, and the more we are able to sense, hear, and feel our biology, the closer we are to our true nature as sensing animals. Silence is everywhere in space, although it's hard to discern sometimes amid the cacophony of the modern soundscape. But remember that silence is the backdrop against which all sound appears.

In Yukti Verse 2 of the Radiance Sutras, Shakti and Shiva continue their conversation about the life force, breath, and sound:

> Radiant One,
> The life essence carries on its play
> Through the pulsing rhythm
> Of outward and inward movement.
> This is the ceaseless throb, the rhythm of life—
> Terrifying in its eternity, exquisite in its constancy.
>
> The inhalation, the return movement of breath,
> Sustains life.
> The outgoing breath
> Purifies life.
> These are the two poles
> Between which respiration goes on unceasingly.
> Between them is every delight you could desire.
>
> Even when the senses are turned outward,
> Your attention on the external world,
> Attend also to the inner throb,
> The pulsing of the creative impulse within you.[1]

EXPLORATION

BREATHING WITH SILENCE

Notice the sound of your breathing and the rate and depth of your inhalation and exhalation as your baseline.

Sounds are all around us, near and far. Tune your hearing to receive the sounds nearby and then those farther in the distance, faint and more subtle. What sounds are in the foreground, the middle ground, and the distance? What may not have been available at first hearing may come to you as you continue to open your sense of hearing.

Listen for the silence behind the sounds, the spaciousness of the silence whose presence is everywhere, including inside us. Move your awareness back and forth between the silence inside and the silence outside. Be simultaneously aware of your breathing and the sound of silence. Attune your breathing to this deep quiet.

Now take time for open attention and take another baseline of the sound of your breathing after this exploration. What have been the rate and depth of your breathing as you've been breathing with silence? Silence can be a resource.

CHAPTER NINETEEN

SWIMMING FOR COHERENCY

The water is your friend. . . . You don't have to fight with water,

just share the same spirit as the water, and it will help you move.

— ALEXANDR POPOV, RUSSIAN SWIMMER, CONSIDERED
ONE OF THE GREATEST SPRINT SWIMMERS IN HISTORY

When I was 15, I tried out for the McBurney School swimming team. I was shy and withdrawn, miserable with my family, and I wanted to be part of something. Football, basketball, and soccer seemed too aggressive to me. I'd been going to the ocean from an early age, so joining the swim team seemed natural.

And it worked. Whenever I was in the pool, though swimming hard to get into shape and prepare for meets, I felt peaceful, held by the enveloping safety of water. I cherished the camaraderie with my teammates, traveling together to schools throughout New York. And perhaps best of all, I would leave home for practice before my parents woke up and then have breakfast with the team before our classes started.

Truth be told, I wasn't all that fast. The only chance I had to compete was to swim butterfly. Most everyone else swam freestyle or backstroke. Even so, I was mostly put on relay teams. When the fastest butterfly swimmer left school, I thought I had a chance; then a younger boy joined the team, and he was faster than I was. Still, I was diligent and earned a varsity letter in my senior year and got to wear an athletic sweater with a big *M* for McBurney on the front.

After college, I joined a masters swimming program. I worked hard, sometimes swimming twice a day before meets, pushing myself to prove I could be good at something. At age 50, I went to the U.S. Masters Swimming National Championships, competing in the 50–54 age range. I was determined to break 30 seconds for the 50-yard butterfly. Most good swimmers can do it in 25 seconds, but it was a personal goal. A friend I swam with every day, Mark, said he said he was going to beat me, and I couldn't let that happen.

When I got up on the starting block for the event, I heard my father's voice say, "You're not going to do it." I looked up toward the sky and replied, "Not today, Dad—get the fuck out of my head." I swam that race in 29-plus seconds and beat Mark, and was in the top 10 in all but one of the seven races I'd entered. Receiving those ribbons was a highlight of my competitive swimming career. And most important, being in the water was always a peaceful time for me. Water was my natural home.

* * *

Soon after I met Emilie Conrad, I told her I'd been swimming and competing since I was 15, and she immediately said, "Stop swimming. You have been patterning your body in that form, and you've lost the ability to be adaptable." I trusted her advice, thinking, *Yes, I'll no longer be swimming in water, but I'm still swimming, this time in my inner waters.* Continuum offered the same peace and quiet, so it felt okay.

Ten years later I had surgery, and afterward I knew I needed to regain strength. So I went back into the water, this time not

competing, counting laps, or timing myself. I swam just for pleasure and form, using my newfound sense of my internal fluidity
to move through the water without stress. I knew that each time
my inner form and swimming form became coherent, my sense
of my body moving through the water was effortless. Each time I
lost my inner fluidity, my swimming got bumpy; the water was no
longer gliding over my body. I would slow down, feel that rough,
uncoordinated place in my body, and bring it back into a coherent
relationship with the rest of my body's movements. These inquiries were based on the principles of Continuum, and the fluid
intelligence within my body showed me the way.

A couple of years ago I was watching men's Olympic gymnas-
tics when one of the men on the U.S. team unexpectedly qualified
for an individual event on the pommel horse, an artistic gymnas-
tics apparatus. He had one jump that he performed in the team
event, but in the individual event he had to show skill in at least
two different routines. He practiced for a number of days to learn a
new form, but he couldn't do it. His body was so patterned in that
one form that he could not find the flexibility to shift.

Emilie taught that the density and the lack of flexibility of
the pelvis create restrictions of movement throughout the body.
In swimming, the rotation of the pelvis creates the power that
drives the arms and legs. Until I "found my pelvis," I was over-
working my arms and rarely kicked. I had no sense of my legs
behind or beneath me. Once I found my pelvis and could rotate it,
my legs came online. All the work I had put into my arms to get
through the water relaxed and came into coordination with my
legs. I kick now.

Knowing how to inhabit my pelvis is a skill I use on dry land
in the standing and sitting postures. Releasing the weight of my
upper body and belly to sit comfortably in my pelvic bowl and
allow my legs underneath to meet the ground, I can also walk
gracefully and fluidly, my breathing supporting the coherency.

Patterns reinforce behavior. Soften the inflexibility of the
body, and we open to innovation and responsiveness. The body is
the vessel of breath, and breath can only move within the shape

of the vessel. When we notice that a patterned posture is limiting our choices and re-creating states that no longer support our present life, it becomes important to change our responses and adapt our shape—and the entry points are movement and breath.

Swimming saved my life. It offered a place I could be with myself and feel the tenderness and welcoming energy of water. Now I swim in a pool and I swim inside myself. Each provides a place of safety that continues to spark my vitality and joy. People ask about breathing while swimming. We breathe in air when part of our face is out of the water, and we exhale while our face is in the water. I'm a much better swimmer today than when I was a teenager, not as fast but smoother and more coordinated. And I still swim butterfly almost every time I go in the water.

While swimming in our neighborhood pool the day before I was to deliver this manuscript to the publisher, I could feel, viscerally, that the wave motions within my body and the wave motions of the pool were the same. When you are in a physical movement that requires muscle activity, the contractions and relaxation activate the water within. In contraction, the water becomes denser as the size of the muscle membrane decreases. When released from contraction, the "water body" sends its wave out into the enlarged container of the relaxed muscle. It's ongoing—waves pulling in and waves fanning out.

Water always reminds me of my wholeness, strength, and endurance. It is a home for my spirit—the spirit that sings when my body can express its fullest potential, when I feel free to be myself, and when my breathing returns to its natural rhythm, which is ease.

EXPLORATION

MOVEMENTS OF
YOUR BREATHABLE BODY

Breathing is a movement process, and breath follows awareness. The air of breath moves through the respiratory system from the tip of the nose to deep in the lungs. All the structures throughout this pathway shape themselves to accommodate the presence of this flow—widening, narrowing, swelling, stretching, expanding, and contracting. These movements are palpable. We have the potential to notice and feel these changes of shape since we have receptors that are part of our nervous system to tell the brain this is happening. The fact that the air touches these receptors allows us to be aware of them through our sense of touch.

The rest of the body that is not in direct contact with the air we breathe also accommodates the flow of breath by moving and changing shape to make room for the changes in shape of the structures of the respiratory system. These movements may be more subtle or less subtle, spreading and receding like the tides of the ocean, a process at once elegantly simple and astoundingly complex. It is this complexity that can keep us engaged in learning and knowing the behavior of a breathable body. The simplicity is in the questions: *Where do I notice movement now, and now, and now, as I breathe in and out?*

At any time, in any position, take a breathing break frequently throughout the day. With eyes open or closed, follow, feel, or sense the movement relationship of breath and body as you inhale and exhale. If you want to receive more movement information, practice *breathing with support* while thinking *Sa~Ha* and placing one or two hands anywhere on your body. The diaphragm; the muscles between the ribs; your face, throat, and chest; and the ribs in the front, along your sides, and in the back (if you can reach them) and the belly will give you the most feedback, as these are the locations in direct relationship with the air of breath. As you get used to inquiring into the movement of your breathable body, you can move your hands or simply your awareness to locations not in direct relationship to the air of breath as well—your extremities, for instance.

Curiosity and interest are all you need. Simply notice. If you practice this for a few months, you may be surprised what you learn about your breathable body and your inner life. You simply need to notice and explore with your awareness and touch.

Knowing and experiencing the movement of your breathable body is a process of becoming more acquainted, familiar, and intimate with this primary aspect of your biology. Keeping a journal of your discoveries deepens the process. Having this kind of awareness can be useful anytime you need to discharge extra energy and support the body in resting.

Welcome home!

CHAPTER TWENTY

TYING IT ALL TOGETHER

The breath of love takes you all the way to infinity.

— RUMI, PERSIAN POET

Breath is a gift that keeps on giving. How many times in life have you been holding your breath during difficult periods, and then when the tide turns, you say with delight, "I can breathe again"? I hope this book has provided that for you—that you can breathe again, that you've become interested in joining with breath on your journey to fullness.

Matt Licata writes: "Underneath the narrative of your life, just below the grand storyline, even beneath the colorful emotional landscape, there exists a rich, mysterious world of sensations—a somatically-organized field of intelligence and creativity. . . . The body is an invitation, an entryway into the freedom, love, and vastness that you are."[1] As the butterfly I encountered in the jungle and wrote about in the Introduction revealed, context and circumstance have everything to do with our breathing. Breath is affected by the life and love around us.

There's an old joke sometimes attributed to Jack Benny: A man arrives in Manhattan with tickets to a classical music concert and gets lost along the way. Then he spots someone looking down on his luck sitting on the sidewalk, and he asks, "Sir, how do you get to Carnegie Hall?" The man looks up and says, in all earnestness, "Practice, practice, practice."

Breathing is the messenger and the message, and it's up to each of us to sense what that means for us. Everything comes and goes, including breath. We can't hold on to a fabulous breath and put it in a box. Like every biological process, breath is constantly changing. I hope you will enter into relationship with your breathable body and transform your world and yourself one breath at a time. Become a sacred activist for personal and planetary wellness. Breathing *with* your whole body sustains your ability to love, and love sustains your desire to breathe. To paraphrase Emilie again, I offer this book to help you fall back in love with your breathing. Thank you for breathing me in. Let us exhale together, awaiting with sacred anticipation our next breath.

EXPLORATION

THE END OF OUR JOURNEY

Be with the movements of your breathable body and let your mind drift as far and wide as it likes while you allow whatever you have learned from our journey together that has been useful for you to rise to the surface of your awareness. Don't go looking; instead, let ideas or images or sensations rise to the surface.

Take your time. Make these your own. They are your keepsakes from our time together. I hope they will become second nature to you, and a leaping-off point for your own unique discoveries. Trust is what is being asked of you, knowing that divine intelligence will point the way. All you need to do is show up and be receptive, engaged, and curious.

APPENDIX A

Benefits of Breathing through Your Nose

Breathing through your nose:

- Warms the incoming air to your body temperature, the optimal temperature for the lungs

- Moisturizes the incoming air, providing the lungs with a liter of water per day

- Filters the incoming air through the hairs and mucous membranes that line the nose to remove particles

- Stimulates secretion of healthy mucus to help keep the airways moist, preventing coughing and throat clearing

- Regulates the velocity and direction of the air stream to maximize exposure to the protective nasal mucosa, whose blanket of cilia provides a protective barrier against bacterial, chemical, and gaseous stimuli

- Keeps your sinus membranes lubricated and functioning well, lessening the chance of stagnation that can lead to sinus infections

- Facilitates the production of nitric oxide, an essential bronchodilator that also sterilizes the air in your sinuses on the way to your lungs

- Triggers the release of immunoglobulins (antibacterial molecules) that help clean the incoming air and improve the functioning of your immune system

- Creates pressure differences between your lungs and nose, assuring the flow of air and oxygen to the heart and lungs

- Imposes a resistance to the flow of air that results in 10 to 20 percent more oxygen uptake, helping maintain the elasticity of the lungs and, ultimately, the function of the heart

- Minimizes loss of carbon dioxide during exhalation, thereby allowing the CO_2 to do its job of reducing constriction in the airways and blood vessels, facilitating the release of oxygen from the red blood cells, and thus maximizing oxygen delivery to the other cells of the body

In addition, breathing through your nose:

- Heightens your sense of smell, linking it to the limbic system—the seat of your emotional body—to allow you to have a clearer sense of how you feel about the things you encounter in your immediate environment

- Maintains your sense of hearing by cleaning the environment around the inner auditory tube at the back of the upper throat to keep it free of stagnating debris

Regular nasal-breathing helps keep the nasal passages open for all the benefits on this list. It also:

- Brings air into your sphenoid sinuses to cool your pituitary gland and help regulate your body temperature

- Regulates sleep by reducing CO_2 emissions, helping keep your nervous and cardiovascular systems' chemistry in balance

- Activates turning the head and body from one side to the other during sleep, ensuring maximum rest and possibly reducing symptoms of backaches, numbness, cramps, and circulatory deficits that can occur from sleeping in only one position

- Activates healthy movement at several head and neck joints—the atlanto-occipital joint, atlantoaxial joint, sphenobasilar joint, and sutures of the facial and head bones—nourishing your central nervous system and helping relax your neck and shoulders

- Moves the air past your nasal septum, slowing the air and facilitating a more complete integration of ventilation with other biological processes

- Provides a clear passageway for tears to drain

- Channels the air past the structures that mark the center of your head, helping keep you balanced and centered

- Reduces snoring

- Stimulates the formation of sinuses in childhood through the movement of air

And last—perhaps most important—breathing through your nose:

- Reduces anxiety by regulating the speed of respiration and encouraging maximum inflation of your lungs, producing a calming effect

- Deepens your connection to yourself and to the present moment by activating your sense of touch as the air passes through your nose and into your lungs (when you're aware of one or more of your senses, you enter deeply into the present moment)

- Facilitates meditation by helping keep you calm and settled, allowing you to tap into your innate sense of well-being

APPENDIX B

PRINCIPLES AND PRACTICES
OF CONTINUUM

In a Continuum class, emergent ideas, potent images, and engaging themes set the groundwork for movement exploration. Different movements are combined with breath and sound to encourage embodied, mindful exploration of each idea, image, or theme. Sitting, standing, or lying down, we change our relationship to gravity to invite new internal feedback and information. The pace of a class may be quiet, slow, and contemplative, with participants exploring barely visible micro-wave movements. A class can also be fast and lively, with a room full of bodies moving in large wavelike, spiraling motions. Continuum fitness classes, called Continuum Playground, combine sound, music, and fluid movement to create aerobic activities using weights and other exercise props and equipment. Classes vary in size from 2 to 50 or more.

Continuum as a regular practice can become part of your daily reality, and many students observe shifts in all the ways they move in the world. The sensibility of Continuum can inform and influence your physical activity, feelings, thoughts, and daily life. Continuum contributes to the field of health and movement education by providing a varied spectrum of movement modalities for all.

For more information, visit www.continuumteachers.com.

APPENDIX C

Five-Day Buteyko Breathing Education Course

When I offer classes on Buteyko Breathing Education, I share the method's principles, science, and practices. Central to the Buteyko Breathing Education is a measurement called the control pause, which involves timing how long you can comfortably hold your breath following an exhalation. According to the Buteyko Clinic International, having a control pause of less than 25 seconds is considered poor, and 25 to 35 seconds means there's room for improvement. The goal is to reach a comfortable breath-hold time of 40 or more seconds. The average control pause of students attending Buteyko clinics worldwide is around 15 seconds. Students attend to help improve their asthma, dysfunctional breathing, anxiety, and sleep problems. With each five-second improvement to their control pause, breathing becomes lighter and the student feels better.[1]

With this in mind, I lead five-day seminars to help quiet and shift breathing behaviors. The coursework and exercises are important, but it's the practice that makes the difference. This means "homework," including journals, records of discoveries, and refinements to my instructions. Knowing how to be in direct contact with the sensations of breath and body will make the process most effective. My first Buteyko teacher, Jennifer Stark, said that the goal is to be able not only to "do" the practices but to "live" them—to incorporate quiet, easy breathing into our lives. In a typical class, students report on their homework and progress, the lesson of the day is presented, practice follows the lesson, questions and responses are next, and homework is assigned. For Buteyko Breathing Education, I have found that having a teacher who can watch your breathing is essential, whether on Zoom or in person.

Here is a typical five-day curriculum:

Day 1

- Principles of Buteyko
- The science of respiration
- The scope of practice
- The value of nasal-breathing
- Nose-clearing exercise
- Clearing reactions (Clearing reactions are times when our breathing improves; and feelings, emotions, and diseases that were earlier suppressed may rise to the surface in order to free breathing from these old restrictions. I described this in Chapter 13, "Asthma," when I had this experience in Mexico City.)
- The meaning of the control pause and how to take one
- First practices in restoring quiet breathing, called by some "reduced breathing," as it is about reducing the volume and pace of breathing from over-breathing to quiet respiration (I have renamed it "restorative breathing," as that is its purpose—to restore and allow breathing that meets our metabolic needs)
- Information for people with asthma and how Buteyko Breathing Education can, under a doctor's supervision, help reduce the need for medications
- How to tape the mouth to facilitate nose-breathing while sleeping

Day 2

- Reporting and sharing of homework and progress
- Continuation of instructions on how to achieve quiet breathing with body-centered practices

- Specific information for asthmatics on how to use the control pause and an extended control pause along with restorative breathing when faced with the need for a rescue inhaler
- Stop-cough exercise
- How to use the control pause to test for foods that might disturb breathing

Day 3

- Reporting and sharing of homework and progress
- Psychological and general symptoms associated with with over-breathing/hyperventilation affecting the respiratory system, nervous system, heart, and teeth, as well as digestion, sleep, and aches and pains
- How to tell the difference between hyperventilation and asthma
- Three breathing exercises to stop hyperventilation episodes and, when needed, asthma: Hyperventilation-Reduction Exercises #1, #2, and #3

Day 4

- Reporting and sharing of homework and progress
- More detailed information about the control pause and its relationship to your breathing health
- Warning signs telling you that your breathing health is deteriorating

Day 5

- Reporting and sharing of homework and progress
- Summing up what has been learned and how to incorporate Buteyko Breathing Education principles and practices into everyday life

- What to do when you get the flu or a chest infection and how to use Buteyko Breathing Education practices to rebuild your breathing health
- Final exercise for coughing, sneezing, yawning, and sighing
- Practicing the mini-pause
- How to talk to your doctors about medications and Buteyko Breathing Education
- Using Buteyko Breathing Education principles and practices for and with physical exercise
- Long-term use of Buteyko Breathing Education principles and practices and how to taper the practices after achieving your goals
- Tips on sleeping well

Each class ends with these reminders:

- Pace yourself so that you can breathe through your nose all day.
- Tape your mouth so you can breathe through your nose all night.
- Take your preventer the way it has been prescribed (for asthmatics).
- Use short-acting reliever medication, as needed (for asthmatics).
- Write down exercises and medication in your workbook.

For more information and listings of Buteyko Breathing Education programs, practitioners, and resources, visit buteykoeducators.org.

APPENDIX D

BUTEYKO BREATHING
EDUCATION EXERCISES

The five practices described here are Buteyko Breathing Education exercises. You can use them along with the "Restorative Breathing" exercise in Appendix G, "Further Explorations," when the need arises. You can also weave them together with the Continuum explorations for greater awareness and effectiveness.

Mini-Pause

Breathe in through your nose, and then exhale through your nose. At the end of the exhale, suspend your breathing for three to five seconds; then resume nasal-breathing. Repeat a few times if needed until you feel a return to quiet breathing and feel your diaphragm and belly being responsive to breathing. (For more about this exercise, see the "Mini-Pause" exploration in Chapter 2, "Your Nose Can Save Your Life.")

Nose Clearing

A stuffed nose can cause you to mouth-breathe, which may activate your sympathetic nervous system and disturb your sleep. For those with high blood pressure and heart issues, please limit yourself to six repetitions of this exercise. For everyone else, you can repeat as often as necessary until you feel a *slight* urge to breathe. It's important to read the instructions all the way through before you try it.

- Breathing through your nose, nod your head slowly backward and forward, allowing gravity to do most of the work. You'll feel a slight drop as your head comes to a natural resting position in back and then in front. (If your nose is too stuffed, then of course breathe through your mouth.)

- Try to relax your neck as your head goes forward, and you'll feel a slight stretch in the muscles at the back of your neck. Never force the movement.

- Breathe smoothly, gently, and as quietly as possible.

- Slowly coordinate the movement of your head with your breathing: Breathe in as your head goes back. Breathe out as your head goes forward. Then, keeping your head upright, take a normal breath in and out through your nose.

- At the end of your exhale, pinch your nostrils closed.

- While holding your breath, tip your head backward and forward three to six times or until you feel a slight urge to breathe. This movement will be faster and more vigorous than before.

- Then release your nostrils and breathe in *very gently* through your nose as if you were trying to receive the subtle odor of a rose.

- Repeat as needed until your nose clears.

If this is uncomfortable for your neck, instead of rocking your head backward and forward, you can stomp your feet as though you are walking, while sitting or standing up. Or you can walk around the room while practicing. It's the *movement* that creates the change.

Three Hyperventilation-Reduction Exercises

Hyperventilation-Reduction Exercise #1

When you practice Hyperventilation-Reduction Exercises #1 and #3, breathe in and out through your nose at whatever rate feels natural and easy to you. There is no need to manipulate your breath to fit a certain rhythm. The same is true for pauses. However long you pause when instructed to do so is fine. When it says "pause for the count of [number]," count in your mind at whatever speed you like. For example, it may take one second or less to pause for the count of two, or it might take three or four seconds.

For this exercise, you go to the count of six and back to settle your nervous system. If you are using it for asthma, you count all the way up to 10 and back. If you are unable to hold your breath that long, in either case, stop and count back from there. You don't want to be so breathless that you have to gasp for breath.

Each time you pause as you go up the scale, the length of time of the pause will change. As you count down from pausing, you can expect that your breathing rate will slow and the pausing for the counts will take longer.

Physiologically, the pausing increases the levels of carbon dioxide, which facilitates the release of oxygen from the blood to the cells and helps you feel rested and settled. You can use this exercise to help you fall asleep or go back to sleep and repeat it until you do so. With every repetition, pause at the end of the second exhale.

- Breathe in and out through your nose twice. Pause for the count of two. Repeat.

- Breathe in and out through your nose twice. Pause for the count of three. Repeat.

- Breathe in and out through your nose twice. Pause for the count of four. Repeat.

- Breathe in and out through your nose twice. Pause for the count of five. Repeat.

- Breathe in and out through your nose twice. Pause for the count of six. Repeat.

- Breathe in and out through your nose twice. Pause for the count of five. Repeat.

- Breathe in and out through your nose twice. Pause for the count of four. Repeat.

- Breathe in and out through your nose twice. Pause for the count of three. Repeat.

- Breathe in and out through your nose twice. Pause for the count of two. Repeat.

- Repeat as needed until you notice that your breathing has settled.

If you want to use this exercise for asthma, you take it up to the count of 10 and then back to the count of 2.

Hyperventilation-Reduction Exercise #2

81 Seconds to Calm Anxiety While Nose-Breathing

The pauses go up to six seconds. You must reverse them when you get to six, and come back down to two.

- Breathe in for two seconds and out for three seconds.
- Pause for two seconds.
- Breathe in for two seconds and out for three seconds.
- Pause for three seconds.
- Breathe in for two seconds and out for three seconds.
- Pause for four seconds.
- Breathe in for two seconds and out for three seconds.
- Pause for five seconds.
- Breathe in for two seconds and out for three seconds.
- Pause for six seconds.

- Breathe in for two seconds and out for three seconds.

- Pause for five seconds.

- Breathe in for two seconds and out for three seconds.

- Pause for four seconds.

- Breathe in for two seconds and out for three seconds.

- Pause for three seconds.

- Breathe in for two seconds and out for three seconds.

- Pause for two seconds.

- Finish, and repeat as needed until you notice that your breathing has settled.

If you want to use this exercise for asthma, you take it up to the count of 10 and then back to the count of 2. This is a good exercise in either case to help someone else who is hyperventilating, since you are directing them each step of the way.

Hyperventilation-Reduction Exercise #3

Nasal-Breathing While Walking

For purposes of anxiety reduction and exercise, follow these instructions until you are holding your breath for 12 to 15 steps. For asthma, do the best you can to get to 20 steps. When you reach the suggested number of steps, start counting down to three or four steps. If at any time the number of steps you take while suspending your breathing feels too difficult, stop at fewer steps, and start counting down to three or four sooner. You can always try again. Over time your endurance may increase, and you may find it easier to walk, do the exercise, and nose-breathe at the same time.

- Breathe in and out through your nose twice while walking. At the end of the second exhale, then suspend your breathing as you continue walking for three or four steps.

- Continue walking, and breathe in and out twice; then suspend your breathing as you continue walking for six or seven steps.

- Continue walking, and breathe in and out twice; then suspend your breathing as you continue walking for nine or ten steps.

- Continue walking, and breathe in and out twice; then suspend your breathing as you continue walking for 12 to 15 steps.

- Continue walking, and breathe in and out twice; then suspend your breathing as you continue walking for nine or ten steps.

- Continue walking, and breathe in and out twice; then suspend your breathing as you continue walking for six or seven steps.

- Continue walking, and breathe in and out twice; then suspend your breathing as you continue walking for three or four steps.

- If using this for an asthma episode, continue increasing the number of steps by two or three each time while suspending your breathing until you get to 20 steps.

- When you reach 12 to 15 steps (or 20 for asthma), decrease the number until you are back to pausing for three or four steps.

- Finish, and repeat as needed until you notice that your breathing has settled.

APPENDIX E

SOME SENSATION WORDS

Sensations are the language of the body. Can you add others to this list?

bloated	bounded	bright	brilliant	bubbly
bumpy	buoyant	burning	burnt	bursting
busting	cold	compacted	compressed	constricted
cool	creaky	crooked	crumbly	crunchy
crusty	damp	dense	drifting	dry
dull	effervescent	elastic	elongated	empty
expanding	expansive	feathery	fiery	flaccid
flat	flexible	floaty	flowing	fluid
fluttery	freezing	full	grabbing	gritty
gushing	hard	heavy	hollow	hot
humid	icy	itchy	jagged	jangled
knotty	leaky	light	limp	little
loose	lumpy	mangled	matted	moist
numb	oozy	opaque	open	packed
penetrating	plump	pointed	poppy	pounding
pressured	pulsating	radiating	raw	rigid
rough	rushing	satiny	scalding	scorching
scratchy	scummy	searing	shallow	sharp
silky	slippery	smooth	snappy	soft
solid	sore	sour	spacious	spreading
square	stretchy	sweaty	sweet	swirling
syrupy	tangled	taught	thick	tickly
tight	tingling	torquing	torrid	turgid
twisted	undulating	vacant	velvety	vibrating
vibrato	voluminous	watery	welling	wet

APPENDIX F

SOME OF THE QUALITIES OF BREATH

continuity	connection	timing	rhythm	pace
volume	phases	cycles	depths	layers
speed	waves	spirals	space	ground
forming	dissolving	unity	sensuous	coherence
resonance	integration	flow	arrival	departure
penetration	transitions	filling	emptying	receptivity
smooth	textured	spacious	softening	tenderness
gentle	beloved	friend	harmony	timelessness
completion	satisfaction	inward	outward	sequencing
wisdom	confidence	security	weight	shape
structure	adventure	endless	known	knowable
unknowable	dependency	love	erotic	forward
back	up/down	humidity	temperature	dimension
emotional	thoughts	feelings	images	silent
musical	harmonious	rising	falling	density
permeable	expansive	intuitive	thoughtful	delicate
inflate	deflate	activated	substantial	relaxed
kindness	energetic	settled	rested	playful
tight	protected	compassion	momentum	ragged
trajectory	shy	organization	tentative	fluid

APPENDIX G

FURTHER EXPLORATIONS

BREATHING *WITH*

In the practice of *breathing with*, we bring to awareness to whatever appears in our mind, body, and heart, including qualities and behaviors of breathing that support our well-being and those that don't. We can do this practice over and over again, and the more we practice it throughout a day, the quicker we'll be able to connect with our breathable body and discover how it responds to breath. We bring attention from the outside environment to our inner landscape, a transformational process. One round of *breathing with* can change our state.

Start with a *baseline*. Become aware of that state of your breathing and your body. What is on your mind and heart? What are the depths and qualities of relationship you are having with your experience?

Inhale through your nose and notice the air entering your nostrils and touching the inner dimensions of your nasal cavity. Notice the temperature, volume, density, rhythm, speed, and texture of your breath. Notice as you inhale if breath expands your body and you feel more spacious and buoyant. Notice on the exhale if you feel more condensed and heavier.

Go slowly. Stay with what you're feeling and experiencing for as long as you remain curious about it. When you begin to lose interest in an area of awareness, move to the next part of the sequence. You can always turn your attention back to an earlier area of the inquiry. Breathe *with* whatever arises in your awareness. Everything you learn about your inner life can be integrated into the ways you move and behave in the world.

As you notice the movements of breath and body, breathe *with* one of these qualities for half a dozen breaths or more—kindness, gentleness, compassion, ease, pleasure, or love—and notice the way your breath and body move with the thought.

Now relax your focus and rest in open attention. This is a time to allow what has been stimulated to organize itself and to integrate what has been revealed. Let whatever comes into your awareness be seen and felt, and then let it pass through. You are learning the mutability of form. Is there a change in the way you perceive yourself or value the process of *breathing with* as a transformational process? A breath partnered with awareness can move you from one state to another. You are learning how to be mindful of your inner world and your actions in the outer world at the same time.

You can also *breathe with* sound, touch, or your own body as you find support in any position. Repeat this sequence one or two more times, if you have the time. Then end with another inquiry, taking note of how you are feeling to compare with your baseline.

We are learning to distinguish states we find easeful from those states that wear us out and dysregulate our nervous system and create anxiety, worry, apprehension, and behavioral patterns that may have served us once but now constrict our vitality. *Breathing with* provides a better understanding of whatever we undertake, including Buteyko Breathing exercises and what they are designed to accomplish.

BEING BREATHED: *SA~HA*

The purpose of this meditation is to compare the way you normally bring air into your body with when you do so using the silent sounds of *Sa~Ha*.

By helping you connect deeply with your internal environment and softening the muscles of your torso, *Sa~Ha* can move you from habitual breathing patterns to a more natural flow, allowing breath to be drawn in by the lungs rather than by your effort. As you become accustomed to this way of breathing, you won't have to use the syllables *Sa* and *Ha* consciously. You will have developed the muscle memory to breathe this way.

Start by taking a baseline, simply noticing the flow and rhythm of your breathing and movements of your breathable body. Observe whatever thoughts, images, feelings, sensations, and memories come into your awareness. There is no right or wrong observation.

If you feel comfortable touching your body, place one hand on your chest and one hand on your belly while you breathe, to get a feeling for where and how your body is responding to breath's movements and the expenditure of energy it takes to breathe.

Most people I work with report that while breathing, they feel some tightening in their head, face, nose, throat, neck, shoulders, chest, or belly. This meditation teaches how to "get out of the way" to allow your body to "breathe you," rather than you breathing your body. You will be bypassing your usual pattern of how you breathe to get a feeling sense of a different way of moving air in and out as your lungs do the breathing. Go slowly. Be kind and gentle with yourself. If at any time this exploration feels uncomfortable or more than you wish to tolerate, stop and do something more pleasant.

Add the silent sound of *Sa* to the process of breathing in, and that of *Ha* to the exhale. *Think* these syllables without making them audible. You hear them in your head, and hearing alters the way the body engages with breathing. Practicing *Sa~Ha* changes how the lungs bring air into the body. Rather than *you* "pulling and releasing" breath, the lungs are actively doing the breathing, bypassing patterned resistances.

Allow your eyes to close (unless you feel better keeping them open). As you inhale, think the syllable *Sa* throughout the length of the inhale. No need to repeat it over and over (*Sa, Sa, Sa*)—just think one long *Sa-a-h*. Then, as the inhale turns into an exhale, think one long *Ha-a-ah* through the length of the exhale. Repeat for a while; then rest and simply notice what may be different from the way you began in your baseline.

With one hand on your chest and one on your belly, now alternate between breathing the way you normally do and breathing while thinking *Sa~Ha*. Take a few breaths one way and a few the other. Go slowly. What do you notice with *Sa~Ha* compared with your usual way of breathing?

Some differences to notice:

- The rhythm and pace of how your body moves with breath

- Where you feel the movement of your body while breathing

- Your current feeling and psychological state

- The effort of your chest muscles
- The effort it takes to breathe
- The sound of your breathing

Anything else? Rest and simply notice.

For the next round, with your hands still on your chest and belly, try to take a really big breath in the way you usually breathe, and notice the tension level in your chest. Then take a big breath while thinking Sa~Ha, and notice the tension levels now. Is there a difference? Rest again and simply notice.

Having your chest muscles tighten when taking a large breath is counterproductive. Tightening limits the capacity of the lungs, making it difficult to take that big breath. When you think Sa~Ha, the chest muscles soften as your lungs draw air into the body. You're "getting out of the way" and allowing the lungs to do the breathing. The lungs know when enough is enough, and by paying attention, you'll get a sense when that happens, bringing satisfaction to your breathing.

Over time, you won't have to think Sa~Ha. As I said before, you'll develop the muscle memory to know how to shift to this way of breathing whenever you sense tension or stress and a need to soften your breathing to return to a balanced, quieter state. You can learn how to breathe this way all day, every day and at night.

While practicing the explorations in this book and in life situations, you can use Sa~Ha and "simply notice" at any time. Some people find it more effective to say, to themselves, "Ha~Sa" rather than "Sa~Ha" as they breathe in and out. Please try it both ways, and see what works for you. You can practice these syllables in either order. This is the beginning of a transformation initiated by breath.

SOUND PRACTICE

Using sound to explore your breathable body facilitates the movement of internal densities, allowing for greater flow and capacity of breathing. Doing sound practice, you may encounter something that until now has been outside of your awareness, awakening parts of yourself to bring them new life.

Pick a position that is comfortable for you, either lying down or sitting. Turn your attention inward and take a baseline by following the flow of breath and the movement of the body in response. Notice how following the movement of your breath and body, you turn your attention from external stimuli to your own inner landscape. Simply notice what you observe, following your awareness wherever it goes.

When you're ready, make a *hum* sound on the exhale that feels and sounds pleasing. Go at a speed that soothes and at a comforting volume and pitch.

While making a hum sound, track how the vibrations (sensations) brought about by the sound travel in your body. You might feel these vibrations anywhere. Without consciously trying to place this sensation anywhere in particular, notice where you feel it now. It will follow its own path.

These vibrations will draw your attention to a particular place. Keep this place in your awareness as you inhale and exhale. Breath follows awareness, so take a moment to sense or feel if this place is being breathed in response to your awareness.

Do this a few more times, or for as long as it feels comfortable and not effortful.

Then stop for a moment of open attention to sense what else might have entered your awareness. After that, take a short baseline to feel if the quality of the inhale has changed as a result of the humming. Is your body more open and responsive as you breathe in and out? Has the effort of breathing changed? Do you have more room to breathe?

Repeat making the sound of *hum* for a few more breaths and notice if the quality of your hum sound has changed. If there is more space and movement with breath, the body may have become a more resonant chamber, shaping the quality and tone of sound, and as a result the hum may change. Be curious.

Note if the vibration goes to a different location or depth when you make the hum sound again. Allow yourself to be surprised by wherever it goes. *Breathe with* wherever the vibration has landed.

Again, stop for a moment of open attention to sense what might be new in your awareness, and then take another short baseline to feel if the quality of the inhale has changed as a result of the humming. Is your body more open and responsive as you breathe in and out? Has the effort of breathing changed? Do you have more room to breathe? Or, if you feel no change at all, or even less room to breathe, note that.

Repeat a third time for a series of six soundings; then go into open attention for a few moments and take yet another baseline to see how you're breathing and the connection you have with your inner world.

- Are there any *natural movements*, micro-movements, arising? Allow yourself to move, if you are so moved. You are becoming familiar with how the inner body speaks to and informs you.

- Are there any thoughts, images, and feelings coming into focus? Simply notice.

- How are you breathing now? How is your breathing capacity? How is the ease of flow? What are the movements of your body in response to breath and sound? Do you feel more awake to yourself and your potential to breathe well?

You can repeat this frequently throughout the day when you need some time to connect to yourself, and especially when you feel your breathing has lost its power to nourish. Or try it once a day to develop the skill of using sound to awaken yourself to your breath. Doing so, you'll gain quicker access to the insights of your inner world and know how to restore movement to your breath—breathing from your whole body. Whole-body breathing can calm your nervous system, and it drops you into recovery mode after anything that may have activated your nervous system.

EXPLORING YOUR TONGUE, LIPS, AND TEETH

The following Continuum explorations can help you become more familiar with the interactive relationship between your tongue, lips, and teeth.

The first is called the "Hum Clock." You'll be using the sound of a hum during this exploration. Try humming to get a feel for it.

Hum Clock

Feel free to close your eyes. That eliminates visual distractions and may enable a greater feeling for what you may be sensing. You'll be using your tongue to feel the variety of textures of your lips and teeth. Do it as a "soft inquiry," probing your lips, teeth, and mouth with your tongue.

Begin by taking a baseline, noticing the textures and spatial arrangements of your mouth, lips, and teeth as well as the flow of your breath. Move your tongue around your mouth to get a better idea of the territory.

Then place your tongue as best you can between the inside of your lips and the front of your teeth and gums. Start at the 12 o'clock position (right below your nose). While resting your tongue there for a moment, gently hum on the exhale. After one cycle of breath while humming, withdraw your tongue back into your mouth's cave; then take a silent breath or two and place your tongue between your lips and front teeth at the 1 o'clock position.

Inhale and then hum while at 1 o'clock. As you move clockwise around your mouth, practice each step (placing your tongue between your lips and teeth, humming, then withdrawing your tongue and taking a couple of breaths before once again moving your tongue out between your lips and the front of your teeth and gums), stopping at each number on the Hum Clock dial until you arrive back at the 12 o'clock position.

When you have reached the 12 o'clock position, repeat each step going counterclockwise until you're back at 12 o'clock again.

Rest and notice the feel of your tongue, lips, and teeth, along with any other information that comes into your awareness. Take time to integrate all that you may have discovered.

The next step is to explore the textures inside the cavity of your mouth. Use your tongue to move about your mouth, surveying the variety of wet, hard, and soft surfaces. Move about randomly. Explore the upper hard and soft palates, the lower palate, and what the tongue feels like in the middle of your mouth. Go slowly to feel your tongue's ability to touch all these surfaces and its relationship to the cavity of your mouth.

Rest when you are ready, and take another baseline while noticing your level of awareness of these structures and your facility with resting your tongue on the roof of your mouth while your lips are lightly touching and your teeth are a few millimeters apart.

Repeating the sequence of any exploration deepens your knowledge and cultivates your innate intelligence. Try doing this practice one to three times and you'll have a new experience of this essential part of you.

Placing your tongue at the roof of your mouth increases your awareness of internal and external environments simultaneously. All your senses seem to benefit, as well as your presence with yourself and your relationship with your environment.

Living in the Kiss

The second exploration is called "Living in the Kiss." I love this exploration; it helps me enjoy keeping my lips lightly sealed.

Lick your lips to moisten them; then let them come together and rest lightly on each other. Can you feel the wetness between them? You are resting your lips on the surface tension of the water between them. This practice helps me remember that we are wet, fluid bodies that can move easily with breath. Throughout the day, I remind myself to nose-breathe and "live in the kiss" while my tongue is nested in the roof of my mouth and my teeth are a few millimeters apart.

Feeling Support:
You Have to Go Down to Go Up

*When you get ready to shoot, make sure your feet are
shoulder-width apart facing the basket and your knees
are bent (much like a spring ready to release). Next, hold the
ball just above your waist lined up to the basket, and all at
once begin your jump, releasing all of your power loaded up
in your bent knees and bent arms at once. Release the ball
at the highest point your hands can go, and keep your
shooting hand pointing at the basket in a straight line.*

— Basketball Coach's Corner, U.S. Sports Camps[1]

We are always supported and grounded by the earth, and we're always in relationship with the space surrounding us and within us. When we feel this, our tensions can relax and release our bracing. Every basketball player knows that to go for a jump shot, you must bend your knees first and get down close to the floor. *You have to go down to go up.*

It's the same with breath. The more the body goes down and feels support during the exhale, the easier it is for the air entering you to lift you up with its buoyancy. This is an exploration to help you discover the ground that's always supporting you.

While you are sitting, standing, or lying down—either on your side, belly, or back with your knees over a pillow or bent so your feet are flat on the floor—turn your attention to the movement of air as it enters through your nose. As air becomes breath, notice your body's responses in movement. (See Chapter 7, "Postures That Support Breath," for more on this topic, including positioning your tongue, lips, and teeth.)

Take a baseline, noticing the feeling of contact with the support beneath, behind, or in front of you and within you. Notice how the outside surface of your body meets the support and how structures within you may be resting on each other. Explore the quality of your breathing—the comfort or effort, how you feel in response to the movement of breath. Where do you feel touched by breath?

Next, practice *Sa~Ha* meditation and allow your lungs to *breathe* you. Do this for half a dozen breaths or more.

Now turn your attention to the force of gravity. As you exhale, your body is being invited down toward the earth. Do you feel heavier? Can you allow your body to yield and receive the support of the surface beneath you?

Like everything else, our bodies are both connected to the ground and lifted into space. We all need support from below; our organs, muscles, and bones rest on structures beneath them. When you feel support from below, what is above can soften, and the lungs can fill more easily. The muscles and bones of your shoulders, for example, can rest on the air in your lungs. Your lungs and heart can rest on your diaphragm. Your belly organs can rest in the pelvis. These are some of the ways the body rests within itself.

Have you ever watched a cat or a dog resting? They're almost magnetically attached to the earth, and their bodies are relaxed, soft, tender, and barely breathing but not short of breath. There's almost no tension in their bodies, so the need for oxygen is reduced.

As you exhale, settle into the support beneath you, and notice the connection between your body and that support. If you're sitting on a chair, feel your sit bones and the chair. If you're lying down, pick one point that is in contact with the support and keep the point of contact in your awareness as you exhale. *You are breathing with support.* Dance between awareness of the buoyancy and the sensation of the weight. This offering of support is without judgment or conditions. It's there to receive you in your fullness.

At the end of each exhale, you may feel even more firmly planted and connected. Or you may find that the support has shifted to a new location. As you inhale, bring this new location of support into awareness. Take your time, and go through at least six cycles of breath, or a period of two to five minutes.

When the body releases some tensions that may have been limiting its breathing capacity, you may notice that the first breath or two after the release can be bigger than normal. The body senses there is more room available to *breathe with* and will take the opportunity to expand more fully. After a few breaths while continuing to be supported, your inhalation will get quieter, increasing the air capacity and recruiting more of your lung tissue to receive air. When you feel complete, go into open attention, allowing new information about your breathable body to come into your awareness. These are lessons learned from the relationship between support and breathing.

Repeat two more times, each round followed by open attention.

As you explore this dynamic, the places you release may surprise you. Over time, you'll probably find that you're releasing tensions from the same places over and over. That's natural. You're learning how you build and rebuild your protective bracing, and you're developing quicker access to and greater facility with softening the protection that may no longer be needed. Your breathing will become more diaphragmatic and easeful, and its capacity will increase.

Take a final baseline and compare it with the baseline you took when you began.

RESTORATIVE BREATHING

This exploration is used in Buteyko Breathing Education to reduce the volume and pace of breaths per minute, to move from over-breathing to quiet, easy respiration—breathing that is "allowed" to find its natural rhythm without manipulation.

Use the postures from Chapter 7, "Postures That Support Breath." Sit in a chair that supports your back and keeps you upright so your chest isn't collapsed over your belly, the horse-rider position. Or you can do this exploration while standing or lying down on your back with your knees supported by a couple of pillows. Your tongue will be at the roof of your mouth with lips slightly touching and teeth in close proximity. Your vision should be peripheral and soft, whether your eyes are open or closed.

Begin by becoming aware of your nasal-breathing. Notice that connecting to the process of breathing immediately shifts its pace. You are already in restorative breathing. Breathe less.

Place one hand on your chest and one hand on your belly so you will be more sensitive to the movements of breathing. Stay with this for five minutes or longer while noticing any subtle changes as you breathe in and out. You are being touched and moved on the inside by breath. Simply notice the touch of the movement of breathing and whatever comes to mind. Breath will follow your awareness and meet the moment with what is needed.

When I practice this exploration, I accommodate the shifts that take place, trusting that whatever I become aware of will guide me to restoring quiet and easy respiration with less volume and less effort.

Allow your nervous system to move from activation to discharge in order to rest and settle. Staying activated all the time without a break makes it difficult to unwind at the end of the day or get a good night's sleep. Learning to unwind, to take a break in the midst of activity, can be nurturing. Settling with your breathing before and after meals and before and after exercise, as well as before sleep, helps you normalize and self-regulate respiration. Restorative breathing is available anytime you need to deactivate your system.

Eventually you'll become proficient at recognizing when you're breathing in a way that brings ease and harmony. During times when you're moving too quickly and breathing feels like a struggle, you can take a nose-breathing break in order to pace yourself and feel balanced and regulated again. Restorative breathing brings you back to vigor, health, strength, and well-being.

BEFRIENDING YOUR BELLY[2]

This is one of my favorite explorations. It involves soft, gentle touch. For some people, this may feel scary and uncomfortable because of emotions that might be associated with your belly. Go slowly so you don't feel overwhelmed. Stay within your window of tolerance, and stop at any time and come back to this exercise later (if you'd like). As you become more intimate with your own breathing belly, I hope you will practice this often. For me, making intimate contact with my belly is a daily practice, relieving any accumulated discomfort. Over time, allowing your belly to breathe freely will, hopefully, become easier.

Day-to-day stress can cause the belly to tighten. Softening your belly can help move the stress through you. You don't need to force your belly to do anything. You don't need to push it out or pull it in. This is an exploration of befriending and inhabiting your belly and opening up the possibilities of movement.

Go to a safe and comfortable space. Privacy is essential, somewhere you know you aren't going to be disturbed. Be gentle with yourself as you venture into the territory of the belly. Go slowly; be kind, curious, and interested; and stop when you feel you've had enough. This is tender territory.

You can start this exploration sitting up. Taking a baseline, pay particular attention to how your belly is responding to breathing in and out. Notice whatever you can, without putting your hands on your body yet.

Before you touch your belly, it's important to befriend your hands. Continuum teacher Cory Blake says, "Your hands are ambassadors of love." Look at your hands and see them as expressions of your heart. You can pour any emotion into your hands, and they can then express that feeling. Imagine them expressing kindness, gentleness, tenderness, and love.

Continue to look at your hands and let your right one, palm down, rest on your left, palm up on your lap, offering support. Take your time until you feel your left hand in a supportive role and your right receiving that support and resting softly on your left hand. When you have a sense of this meeting of hands, reverse them so that right hand is now receiving support while the left, below, is offering it. Your hands are making friends with each other.

Now let the right hand explore the left hand—its shapes, textures, temperature, and features. Allow the right hand to have an attitude of curiosity and caring. Take your time; there is a lot of surface to explore—the front of the hand and the back, the fingers and the spaces between them, the bones deep in your palm, the soft tissue, and the textures of the skin. Be imaginative in how you learn about your left hand. Try making a pleasurable sound: a hum, a "yum," or some other tender vocalization. This may deepen your interest in the complexity of your left hand. Gently squeeze your left hand with your right. Do anything you can that might make you more aware of your left hand.

When you feel you are finished, take a moment for open attention. Sit, breathe, and notice the quality of awareness in your hands, their relationship to each other and to the rest of your body, the feeling in your belly and your heart, and the rhythm and depth of your breathing.

Now let the left hand explore the right hand—its shapes, textures, temperature, and features. Remember to be aware of how your belly is breathing as you do this. Your belly already knows that your hands will eventually be moving toward it. If the touch is rough, your belly will tighten and not breathe well. If your touch expresses interest and love, your belly will respond in kind. When you are done, go into open attention, sensing your hands and how they fit with your body and how your belly is breathing.

At this point you can remain seated or lie down, preferably on your back with your knees bent or over a pillow, maybe with a small pillow under your head or neck. Stay as comfortable and warm in this position as possible. When you're ready, begin to approach your belly slowly with your hands, taking as long as necessary, stopping along the way at any point when you feel you can't get any closer. Wait there until you feel safe enough to continue. If this is as far as you can get, that's okay. Stop here and let this be enough for now. You can always come back to this exploration again and again.

If you can go on, continue to approach your belly slowly until both hands are surrounding your navel. Remember to envision your hands as ambassadors of love.

As soon as your hands land lightly on your belly, let them rest there. Take the time you need to allow your belly and your whole organism to adjust to their presence. In resting your hands there, you are inviting your belly to be the support for your hands. Give your belly and the rest of your body time to organize this support, and get used to the idea that, in this moment, that is their only task. Give your belly time to trust that you have no other agenda. Your hands stay passive and at the same time attentive and curious. It's okay if this is all you do for this exploration. Introducing your hands to your belly might be enough for today.

The first time I did this exploration with Susan Harper, it took 20 minutes for my belly to soften and trust my hands and for my hands to be interested in my belly. I felt like a genuine meeting was taking place. My hands and my belly were in relationship to each other.

If you continue, begin to bring your hands' attention to your belly's movements as seamlessly as possible as you breathe in and out. Just follow the movement, breath by breath. Take as long as needed to feel the relationship between your hands and your breathing belly, continuing to develop a deepening of trust and comfort. Don't ask your belly to "be" any special way; just observe with your hands how it moves when you breathe.

If you don't find comfort through this exploration or it starts to feel *un*comfortable, stop. Remove your hands, feel the support beneath your body, and let your mind go into open attention. If feelings are coming up, allow in as much as you can, or if it's too uncomfortable, get up and find something to do that pleases you. Remember, stay in your window of tolerance. Trust yourself to know what is good for you, and perhaps, over time, that window of tolerance may change.

When you get to the point where you sense that your belly trusts your hands and your hands are receiving the movement of your belly while breathing, rest for a moment in this partnership. This may be all you do for now. The meeting is the essential step.

If you feel comfortable continuing, then allow your hands to be gently active in touch and explore the size, shape, textures, and layers of the belly's tissues. Go very slowly and tenderly. Feel how your hands might caress or massage your belly, with the idea that this may help it soften and be more breathable. You are not doing this to *make* your belly more breathable. The movement of your hands is an invitation, not a command. If your hands start to feel too invasive and your belly is resisting, pause and rest in open attention. Just notice how the belly is breathing and how the rest of the body breathes when you have more awareness of your belly.

If you have time and want to do another round, explore your hands again one at a time, as you did before. You can stay lying down with your hands lifted in front of you. Notice how each might feel different this time. Take time for open attention before changing the focus to the other hand. Then repeat the sequence of approaching and making a relationship with your belly.

If you have time and want to do a third round, it can help increase your awareness of your breathing belly and your body breathing. If you don't have time or don't feel inclined to do more today, come back to it later. The trust that was built this first time will be a source of support.

If you want to explore this further, I suggest Allison Post and Stephen Cavaliere's book *Unwinding the Belly* (see "Further Reading" in the closing pages of this book). It offers specific ways to touch your belly that help release tensions. Trust your intuition as you develop an intimate relationship with your belly, touching it in ways that feel comforting and loving.

APPENDIX H

Frequently Asked Questions

I receive a variety of questions from students, clients, and those who attend workshops, and my responses are always from a breathing perspective. Of these questions and my responses, I am sharing 16 of them here.

1. Why do we yawn?

2. What about sighing?

3. What about teeth grinding, jaw clenching, and breathing?

4. What about frequent burping and gas?

5. Why do I need to clear my throat so often?

6. How do I stop my cough?

7. Why is it that when I practice quiet breathing, my salivary glands get more active and my eyes water?

8. Can I nose-breathe while exercising? Why is breath holding effective in boosting athletic performance, facilitating recovery from long COVID, and promoting general health?

9. What is carbon dioxide tolerance?

10. What are the benefits of diaphragmatic breathing?

11. What is reverse breathing?

12. Do I nose-breathe during lovemaking?

13. Is over-breathing related to overeating?

14. What about nitric oxide and humming?

15. What about talking and breathing? Don't we use our mouths to talk?

16. What about breathing while singing?

This is not medical advice. If any of the conditions in question pertain to you, especially if they're chronic or disturbing, please seek medical advice. I hope my perspective can add to your treatment plan in a complementary fashion.

Why do we yawn?

Yawning helps bring in more oxygen. It is involuntary and circumstance related. When you've been active or gone through a period of stress, yawning may follow. It can be "contagious." Even thinking about it can start the yawning process. A new theory suggests that yawning helps cool the brain.[1]

Chronic yawning—when you yawn throughout the day—is a form of over-breathing, since you're continually using your mouth to breathe. It has underlying causes that need to be addressed. If this is the case for you, it would be wise to visit a health practitioner. MedlinePlus, an information service of the U.S. National Library of Medicine, has information on excessive yawning.[2]

When I'm working with someone who yawns chronically, the first thing I teach them is to yawn with their mouth closed. This stops over-breathing, which releases too much carbon dioxide and reduces the distribution of oxygen to the cells for energy production.

For those with allergies, asthma, COPD, emphysema, anxiety or panic disorders, digestive challenges, or high blood pressure, I also suggest that they yawn with their mouths closed, minimizing the symptoms of over-breathing. For those who do not have these challenges, I recommend that they yawn, settle, and return to normal nasal-breathing.

What about sighing?

Sighing is usually an open-mouthed exhale. It's generally a sigh of relief, but it can also be an expression of overwhelm, stress, sadness, or grief. People with respiratory challenges like asthma and COPD also tend to sigh more.

Sighing can serve a healthy function for the lungs. Sometimes the alveoli (the small air sacs in the lungs) may collapse from under-breathing (hypoventilation or shallow breathing), and sighing signals the brain to take a deeper breath to reinflate them.

Sighing can be involuntary. Healthline reports that humans, on average, produce 12 spontaneous sighs an hour.[3]

What about teeth grinding, jaw clenching, and breathing?

Bruxism is a condition in which you grind, gnash, or clench your teeth. If you have bruxism, you may unconsciously clench your teeth when you're awake or grind them when you're asleep.[4]

Breathing is meant to be easeful, silent, and slow, with the diaphragm and belly active but relaxed. When we're rested, settled, and relaxed, breath slides through the airways with little restriction. When the airway decreases in size, the effort in breathing increases, a bigger airway needed just at the time when there's less room. Teeth grinding and jaw clenching may be efforts to find more room. In the long term, clenching and grinding can crack the teeth and degrade the temporomandibular joint, the hinge that connects the lower jaw to the skull, located in front of each ear.

Many studies posit a correlation between bruxism and breathing. One shows an association between bruxism, respiratory problems such as asthma and airway infections, and dental cavities in young children.[5] Another indicates a significant relationship between bruxism, clenching, and airway problems with oxygen desaturation and the lowering of pH in the esophagus, which goes along with sleep apnea.[6] In a sleep-apnea event, when the body is not getting enough air, the fight-or-flight response creates further tension in the chewing muscles.

What about frequent burping and gas?

These are generally the result of too much air in the digestive tract. You may be mouth-breathing and swallowing too much air while you inhale, which leads to poor digestion and the buildup of the gases. A release of gas through belching or passing wind might not happen until the body is in a state of relaxation and the buildup is ready to be released. That may be a sign that you've been stressed and are now settling.

Why do I need to clear my throat so often?

Mouth-breathing can dry out the air passageways, causing them to feel irritated. This, in turn, may generate increased mucus production to moisten the airways. Clearing your throat may be an attempt to move mucus and other irritants out of the airway.

According to the University of Kentucky News, "In general, chronic throat clearing is usually the result of hypersensitivity in the larynx (voice box) and pharynx (throat). Clearing your throat is usually your body's response to this irritation and an effort to remove the irritation by rubbing your vocal folds (vocal cords) together. Chronic throat clearing often creates more irritation to the vocal folds because of the harsh contact, resulting in a cycle of frequent persistent throat clearing."[7]

Clients and students who have come to me have found relief from throat clearing by staying hydrated and becoming a more ardent nose breather. I have observed that often throat clearing arrives after episodes of mouth-breathing and talking and taking big breaths in between sentences. If you do clear your throat, do it as gently as possible so as not to irritate your vocal cords.

How do I stop my cough?

There can be many factors causing your cough, including acid reflux, postnasal drip from allergies or sinusitis, vocal-cord lesions, neurological conditions such as tics, and side effects from medications. As soon as you begin to cough or feel you are about to cough, put your hand over your mouth (this stops you from taking a big breath in through your mouth). Swallow once and take a small breath in and out through your nose.

Hold your breath for a few seconds. Then breathe in and out slowly and smoothly for at least 30 seconds, with your hand still over your mouth. Now tell yourself that you're not going to cough. Take a smooth, normal breath through your nose; then take your hand away from your mouth. If you still feel a tickle, repeat the exercise.

Why is it that when I practice quiet breathing, my salivary glands get more active and my eyes water?

When your body relaxes due to the quiet breathing, your nervous system goes into "rest, settle, and digest." Salivation is part of the digestive process, so more saliva is produced even if you're not eating. Saliva keeps the tongue and gums moist and protects against gum disease, tooth decay, and oral infections. It helps reduce microbial buildup on the teeth by producing agents that kill or inhibit the growth of microorganisms such as bacteria and fungi. It also helps eliminate bad breath caused by a buildup of bacteria.

Watering eyes is another sign that the body is de-stressing and may accompany quiet breathing, a yawn, or a sigh.

Can I nose-breathe while exercising? Why is breath holding effective in boosting athletic performance, facilitating recovery from long COVID, and promoting general health?

In yoga, the practice of breath retention, called *kumbhaka*, has been used for centuries. Many masters say that it can result in greater health and enhanced stamina, and scientific findings are corroborating this. During breath retention, our spleen contracts, releasing blood rich in oxygen-carrying red blood cells. We also experience a release of erythropoietin, a hormone that increases the red blood cell count and the efficiency of mitochondria.

A conscious breath hold can build the body's capacity to transport and utilize more oxygen, and can be a powerful tool for enhancing athletic performance. Altitude training is based on similar principles. Being in a low-oxygen zone forces our body to adapt by increasing red blood cell production to carry more oxygen. That way after returning to sea level, we can enjoy the benefits of increased performance. Breath holding simulates that kind of environment.

Exhale-hold or altitude-simulation techniques can be used to drop the oxygen saturation in your body, if only for a moment. As part of a training program, even these short moments can build up a meaningful advantage. Breath retention is a complex technique, and if you wish to try it, I always recommend that you learn it with a qualified teacher. Your teacher will show you how to perform a maximum breath hold after a light exhalation (leaving 30 to 40 percent of the air in your lungs). For safe and effective training, your teacher should use a pulse oximeter to monitor your oxygen levels.

In addition to practicing breath holding with a qualified teacher, you can learn more about this process from an Oxygen Advantage practitioner or by reading *The Oxygen Advantage* by Patrick McKeown.

What is carbon dioxide tolerance?

Carbon dioxide tolerance is the amount of carbon dioxide that your respiratory center can tolerate before it initiates an inhale. The lower the tolerance, the faster the breathing rate. Low tolerance of carbon dioxide can lead to feeling suffocated and anxious if you involuntarily hold your breath, causing CO_2 levels to rise beyond your tolerance. It is also one of the reasons why people with a low tolerance for CO_2 have trouble wearing masks. The levels of CO_2 in your blood regulate its acid–base balance, determining the ease of the flow of oxygen from the blood to the cells for energy production.

Having the optimal tolerance for CO_2 is one of the most significant things that you can do for your mental, physical, and emotional health. Finding a practitioner who uses a CapnoTrainer to calculate end-tidal CO_2 levels at the end of your exhale is a way of measuring your tolerance. The Buteyko Breathing Education control pause is another way of measuring carbon dioxide tolerance. We often think of CO_2 as negative, a by-product that we have to get rid of. Carbon dioxide also plays an important role in our body as a vasodilator and bronchodilator, increasing the dimensions of our vessels and airways.

What are the benefits of diaphragmatic breathing?

Compared with shallow chest breathing, diaphragmatic breathing is more relaxing and makes the process of gas exchange more efficient. You are using your primary breathing muscle rather than experiencing the stress of using secondary breathing muscles. The oxidative stress caused by mental or physical exhaustion can be mitigated by diaphragmatic breathing. You may have heard that good breathing practices can enhance the immune system, and there's some truth to this. Diaphragmatic breathing helps move the lymph, and therefore pathogens, through the lymph nodes, where they can be treated with specific lymphocytes. Another benefit is increased blood flow to the heart. Finally, if you strengthen the diaphragm as a muscle (through regular diaphragmatic breathing), you'll increase your endurance.

What is reverse breathing?

Reverse breathing is a biomechanical, dysfunctional way to breathe, setting up chest breathing and signaling the body to create an activated state. The normal movement of the diaphragm on inhaling is downward toward the belly, and the belly moves outward without pushing. On the exhale, the diaphragm moves upward toward the lungs, and the belly flattens.

Reverse breathing is the opposite. In reverse breathing, the lung space is made smaller, reducing its capacity. It feels more like chest breathing. I have a client who pushes her belly out while, at the same time, reverse breathes using her stomach muscles to pull her stomach inward and upward, preventing the diaphragm from moving in its designed functioning.

Here is one way you can tell you are reverse breathing. Place your hands on you belly and chest as you breathe in and out. If your belly moves outward without pushing it out on the inhale and withdraws toward your spine as you exhale the diaphragm is moving in, this is "normal." If the opposite happens—you find that you're pulling your belly inward and upward while inhaling and downward out outward while exhaling—you are reverse breathing.

There is a practice in some martial arts, also called reverse breathing, of expanding the abdomen while breathing out through the nose and then compressing it while inhaling through the mouth. I am not commenting on this practice. I am talking about a pattern that is unintentional and does not serve the individual caught in it. If you think you might be reverse breathing, I recommend seeing a breathing coach who can help you become more aware of the pattern, the ways it doesn't serve you, and how to shift if, over time, with practice.

Do I nose-breathe during lovemaking?

Nose-breathing creates a circulation of energy, building passion. The nose keeps the fire of passion within the body, rather than being dissipated by mouth-breathing. The moment of orgasm is the time for the release of that fire that includes an open-mouthed expression of joy. Then return to nose-breathing to harvest the glow.

Is over-breathing related to overeating?

As a member of Weight Watchers, I learned about portion size. As I reported earlier, for many years I had trouble maintaining a weight that felt like I was living in a body that moved well and was healthy. I would slide up and down the scale, give or take 30 pounds. Each time I reached that delicious place of feeling good, the next day I started gaining weight. I was too afraid to live in my body comfortably.

Over the years in my Buteyko Breathing Education practice, I've seen a significant correlation between over-breathing and overeating, and I've heard this from Buteyko colleagues as well. And I've observed that when some of my clients stopped over-breathing, they also stopped overeating. That has had a significant impact on me as well, and I've maintained a comfortable weight for many years now without trying. Perhaps the need for less breath to feel satisfied translates to needing less food to feel satisfied.

When I feel I'm not getting the nourishment I want, I ask myself what I really need in that moment. Sometimes it's food. At other times it's liquid; I'm thirsty. At times it's the need to slow down and regulate my breathing. At still other times, it's a need to rest and relax or to take a walk in nature. And sometimes it's co-regulation with another person, a conversation, or just being together. All of these things help settle my breathing.

Try to notice whether over-breathing less changes how you approach food.

What about nitric oxide and humming?

Nitric oxide (NO) is a highly effective vasodilator (it helps relax blood vessels) and antifungal, antiviral, and antibacterial molecule. One study showed that humming for 20 minutes a day increases the production of NO by 15 to 20 times.[8]

NO is produced in nearly every type of cell in the body, including in the paranasal sinuses, from which it's excreted into the nasal airways. It has been used exogenously (from outside the body) with COVID-19 patients to help reduce their viral load.

What about talking and breathing? Don't we use our mouths to talk?

Yes, of course we do. Talking is making sounds; it's "audible breath." While expressing ourselves with language or sounds, we're exhaling. To get more air/breath to continue talking, we have to inhale. In that stage of the breathing cycle, we have a choice.

Following the principle of *pacing your breathing to your activity level*, how, then, do you inhale? Inhaling through your nose is the best option to settle yourself while talking. Remember that breathing with your mouth activates your sympathetic nervous system. Repeatedly inhaling through the mouth escalates the activation, and you can lose your train of thought. Stop talking when you sense you're running out of breath while speaking. You can pause and take a moment to breathe with your nose.

Throughout this book you've practiced explorations and exercises designed to give you a felt sense of the experience of breathing. This is what is needed when talking. You can pause for a moment while you turn your attention to your breathable body, to your breathing and your body's response—a moment with yourself, for yourself. Your attention in that moment is focused on your breathing experience.

When satiated by the inhale, you begin talking again, trusting you will pick up the conversation where you left off, not only reengaging but doing so with more presence. You have given yourself a moment of attention, and now you have energy for the other person or people.

If you gesture with your hand that you wish to pause for a moment, or if your listener knows you, they can take a pause while you're in a pause, perhaps processing and integrating the last thing you said. Now when you speak again, they have more capacity to hear and absorb your next words.

Practicing this, of course, can be awkward. A way to learn how to do this is to read aloud and use commas and periods as natural breath pauses. Not every comma but ones that break up long sentences. William Shakespeare annotated his plays with breath pauses to give the actors a break. Speaking this way is another lesson in patience, timing, and receiving your felt-sense experience.

I went to a lecture where the woman was speaking and mouth-breathing so fast that I said to myself, *She is going to start falling apart soon.* About a half hour into her talk, she was forgetting what she wanted to say. After the lecture, I went up to her and brazenly pointed this out. She was a bit incensed and wanted to know who I was and on what authority I could say this. I told her my credentials as a breathing educator. About an hour later, after an informal gathering with snacks, she came up to me and told me she had been practicing nose-breathing since our talk and felt much more relaxed. She was impressed by what a difference it made. That experience actually led me to be invited to teach Buteyko Breathing Education to visiting doctors at the Andrew Weil Center for Integrative Medicine at the University of Arizona.

What about breathing while singing?

Singers have expressed difficulty in being able to nose-breathe the way I suggest. They say that the phrases they sing are too quick for a pause, they need a quick breath, and getting it through their mouths is easiest. Some songs actually allow more space, making it possible to pause and breathe.

Since the singers who have come to me have breathing challenges (mostly asthmatics), my suggestion is to settle their breathing before the performance and then to restore it afterward so they don't go on breathing in a dysregulated way. If there is an instrumental riff, for example, and they're not singing for a while, that's also a good time to settle their breathing.

FURTHER READING

David Abram, *The Spell of the Sensuous: Perception and Language in a More-Than-Human World* (New York: Vintage, 1997)

Judith Blackstone, *Trauma and the Unbound Body: The Healing Power of Fundamental Consciousness* (Boulder, CO: Sounds True, 2018)

Janet Brindley, *Breathe Well and Live Well with COPD* (London: Singing Dragon, 2014)

Michael J. Cohen, *Reconnecting with Nature: Finding Wellness through Restoring Your Bond with the Earth* (Corvallis, OR: Ecopress, 2007)

Elaine Colandrea and Rori Smith, *The Elemental Body: A Movement Guide to Kinship with Ourselves and the Natural World* (Rhinebeck, NY: Epigraph, 2022)

Emilie Conrad, *Life on Land: The Story of Continuum, the World-Renowned Self-Discovery and Movement Method* (Berkeley, CA: North Atlantic Books, 2007)

Saundra Dalton-Smith, *Sacred Rest: Recover Your Life, Renew Your Energy, Restore Your Sanity* (Nashville, TN: FathWords/Hachette, 2017)

Antonio Damasio, *The Feeling of What Happens: Body and Emotion in the Making of Consciousness* (New York: Mariner Books, 2000)

Deb Dana, *The Polyvagal Theory in Therapy: Engaging the Rhythm of Regulation* (New York: W. W. Norton, 2018)

Peter Francis Dziuban, *Simply Notice: Clear Awareness Is the Key to Happiness, Love and Freedom* (self-pub., 2017)

Clarissa Pinkola Estés, *Women Who Run with the Wolves: Myths and Stories of the Wild Woman Archetype* (New York: Ballantine Books, 1996)

Donna Farhi, *The Breathing Book: Good Health and Vitality through Essential Breath Work* (New York: Henry Holt, 1996)

———, *When You Breathe*, illus. Billy Renkl (New York: Abrams Books, 2020)

Bonnie Gintis, *Engaging the Movement of Life: Exploring Health and Embodiment through Osteopathy and Continuum* (Berkeley, CA: North Atlantic Books, 2007)

David Gorman, *The Body Moveable: Blueprints of the Human Musculoskeletal System—Its Structure, Mechanics, Locomotor, and Postural Function* (Guelph, ON: Ampersand Press, 1981)

Alexis Pauline Gumbs, *Undrowned: Black Feminist Lessons from Marine Mammals* (Oakland, CA: AK Press, 2020)

François Haas and Sheila Sperber Haas, *The Chronic Bronchitis and Emphysema Handbook* (Hoboken, NJ: John Wiley & Sons, 2000)

Teresa Hale, *Breathing Free: The Revolutionary 5-Day Program to Heal Asthma, Emphysema, Bronchitis, and Other Respiratory Ailments* (New York: Three Rivers Press, 2000)

Hans Jenny, *Cymatics: A Study of Wave Phenomena and Vibration* (Eliot, ME: MACROmedia Publishing, 2001)

Jon Kabat-Zinn, *Mindfulness Meditation for Pain Relief: Practices to Reclaim Your Body and Your Life* (Boulder, CO: Sounds True, 2023)

Ron Kurtz, *Body-Centered Psychotherapy: The Hakomi Method* (Mendocino, CA: LifeRhythm, 1990)

Peter A. Levine: *Waking the Tiger: Healing Trauma* (Berkeley, CA: North Atlantic Books, 1997)

Matt Licata, *A Healing Space: Befriending Ourselves in Difficult Times* (Boulder, CO: Sounds True, 2020)

Peter M. Litchfield and Sandra Reamer, *Learn to Screen Clients for Dysfunctional Breathing Habits: Are Breathing Mechanics Aligned with Respiratory Chemistry?* (Cheyenne, WY: Professional School of Behavioral Health Sciences, 2019)

Gabor Maté, *When the Body Says No: Understanding the Stress-Disease Connection* (Hoboken, NJ: John Wiley & Sons, 2011)

Gabor Maté with Aaron Maté, *The Myth of Normal: Trauma, Illness & Healing in a Toxic Culture* (New York: Avery/Penguin Random House, 2022)

Patrick McKeown, *Anxiety Free: Stop Worrying and Quieten Your Mind* (Moycullen, Ireland: Buteyko Books, 2010)

———, *Close Your Mouth: Buteyko Clinic Handbook for Perfect Health* (East Sussex, U.K.: Gardners Books, 2003)

———, *Sleep with Buteyko: Stop Snoring, Sleep Apnea and Insomnia, Suitable for Children and Adults* (Moycullen, Ireland: Buteyko Books, 2011)

———, *The Oxygen Advantage: The Simple, Scientifically Proven Breathing Techniques for a Healthier, Slimmer, Faster and Fitter You* (New York: William Morrow, 2015)

Thomas W. Myers, *Anatomy Trains: Myofascial Meridians for Manual Therapists and Movement Professionals* (Amsterdam: Elsevier, 4th ed., 2020)

James Nestor, *Breath: The New Science of a Lost Art* (New York: Penguin, 2021)

Frank H. Netter, *Atlas of Human Anatomy* (Amsterdam: Elsevier, 7th ed., 2018)

Stephen W. Porges, *The Pocket Guide to the Polyvagal Theory: The Transformative Power of Feeling Safe* (New York: W. W. Norton, 2017)

Allison Post and Stephen Cavaliere, *Unwinding the Belly: Healing with Gentle Touch* (Berkeley, CA: North Atlantic Books, 2003)

Swami Rama, Rudolph Ballentine, and Alan Hymes, *Science of Breath: A Practical Guide* (Honesdale, PA: Himalayan Institute Press, 1996)

Reginald A. Ray, *Touching Enlightenment: Finding Realization in the Body* (Boulder, CO: Sounds True, 2008)

Beth Pettengill Riley and Priscilla Stanton Auchincloss, *A Moving Inquiry: The Art of Personal Practice* (Rhinebeck, NY: Epigraph, 2019)

Lorin Roche, *The Radiance Sutras: 112 Gateways to the Yoga of Wonder and Delight* (Boulder, CO: Sounds True, 2014)

Theodor Schwenk, *Sensitive Chaos: The Creation of Flowing Forms in Water and Air* (East Sussex, U.K.: Rudolf Steiner Press, 2014)

Laura Sewall, *Sight and Sensibility: The Ecopsychology of Perception* (Los Angeles: Jeremy Tarcher, 1999)

Jennifer Stark and Russell Stark, *The Carbon Dioxide Syndrome* (Moycullen, Ireland: Buteyko Online, 2002)

Don St John, *Healing the Wounds of Childhood: A Psychologist's Journey and Discoveries from Wretched Beginnings to a Thriving Life* (Salt Lake City: Paths of Connection, 2015)

David Suzuki, *The Sacred Balance: Discovering Our Place in Nature* (Vancouver, BC: Greystone Books, 2007)

Eckhart Tolle, *The Power of Now: A Guide to Spiritual Enlightenment* (Novato, CA: New World Library, 2004)

Bessel van der Kolk, *The Body Keeps the Score: Brain, Mind, and Body in the Healing of Trauma* (New York: Penguin Publishing Group, 2015)

Matthew Walker, *Why We Sleep: Unlocking the Power of Sleep and Dreams* (New York: Scribner, 2018)

Sharon Weil, *ChangeAbility: How Artists, Activists, and Awakeners Navigate Change* (Los Angeles: Archer/Rare Bird, 2018)

ONLINE RESOURCES

Better Physiology Ltd.: betterphysiology.com

Breathe Your Truth: breatheyourtruth.com

Buteyko Breathing Educators Association: buteykoeducators.org

Buteyko Institute of Breathing & Health: buteyko.info

Continuum Teachers Association: www.continuumteachers.com

Rosalba Courtney, Integrative Breathing Therapy: www.rosalbacourtney.com

Robert Litman, The Breathable Body: thebreathablebody.com

Robert Litman (audio), Breathing for Better Health: Exercises & Meditations. www.hayhouse.com/breathing-for-better-health-exercises-meditations-audio-download

Robert Litman YouTube Channels: www.youtube.com/@rtl1944 and www.youtube.com/@ThebreathablebodyVashon

ENDNOTES

1. Lorin Roche, *The Radiance Sutras: 112 Gateways to the Yoga of Wonder and Delight* (Boulder, CO: Sounds True, 2014), 36.

My Journey with Breath: An Introduction

1. Roche, *The Radiance Sutras*, 166.

PART I: THE BREATH OF LIFE

1. Adapted from *The Complete Jewish Bible*. See https://www.biblestudytools.com/genesis/2-7-compare.html.

Chapter One: Breathing *With*

1. Matt Licata, Facebook Post (January 23, 2016, https://m.facebook.com/mattlicataphd/posts/underneath-the-narrative-of-your-life-just-below-the-grand-storyline-even-beneat/1503218806652001/)

2. Matt Licata, "On Therapy," from his blog *A Healing Space . . . reflections on love, meaning, and the aliveness of immediate experience* (December 11, 2020, http://alovinghealingspace.blogspot.com/2020/12/on-therapy.html).

3. Eckhart Tolle, *Stillness Speaks* (Novato, CA: New World Library, 2003), 31.

4. Eckhart Tolle, *The Power of Now: A Guide to Spiritual Enlightenment* (Novato, CA: New World Library, 2004), 49.

5. See Peter Francis Dziuban, *Simply Notice: Clear Awareness is the Key to Happiness, Love and Freedom.* (Carlsbad, CA: Balboa Press, 2013).

Chapter Two: Your Nose Can Save Your Life

1. Andrew Benner et al, "Physiology, Bohr Effect" *National Library of Medicine* (August 8, 2022) https://www.ncbi.nlm.nih.gov/books/NBK526028.

2. See, e.g., Erica Cirino, "Empty Nose Syndrome," *Healthline*, updated August 15, 2018, https://www.healthline.com/health/empty-nose-syndrome#causes; and Edward C. Kuan, Jeffrey D. Suh, and Marilene B. Wang, "Empty Nose Syndrome," *Current Allergy and Asthma Reports* 15, no. 1 (January 2015), https://pubmed.ncbi.nlm.nih.gov/25430954.

3. See "How Long Does It Take to Form a Habit?," *University College of London News*, August 4, 2009, https://www.ucl.ac.uk/news/2009/aug/how-long-does-it-take-form-habit; and "How Long Does It Take for a New Behavior to Become Automatic?," *Healthline*, reviewed October 24, 2019, https://www.healthline.com/health/how-long-does-it-take-to-form-a-habit#base-figure.

Chapter Three: The Sensuous Nature of Breathing

1. From Emilie Conrad, "Continuum Movement," in New Dimensions in Body Psychotherapy, ed. Nick Totton (Berkshire, U.K.: Open University Press, 2005), 142–52.

2. Sophia Reinders, "The Sensuous Kinship of Body and Earth," *Ecopsychology* 9, no. 1 (March 1, 2017), https://doi.org/10.1089/eco.2016.0035.

3. Michael J. Cohen, *Reconnecting with Nature: Finding Wellness through Restoring Your Bond with the Earth* (Corvallis, OR: Ecopress, 2007), 50. Italics added.

Chapter Four: Continuum and the Fluidity of the Breathable Body

1. Emilie Conrad, "Continuum Movement," *USA Body Psychotherapy Journal* 4, no. 1(2005), 29–34, https://ibpj.org/issues/usabpj-articles/(3)_Conrad__E._ Continuum_Movement._USABPJ_4.1__2005.pdf.

2. Thanks to Ajaya Sommers for the wording of this paragraph (https:// ajayasommers.com).

3. Emilie Conrad Da'Oud, "Life on Land," in Don Hanlon Johnson, ed., *Bone, Breath, and Gesture: Practices of Embodiment* (Berkeley, CA: North Atlantic Books, 1995), 307.

4. Greg Wilson, "Cheetahs on the Edge—Director's Cut," Vimeo video, 7:07, uploaded November 19, 2012, https://vimeo.com/53914149?cjevent=a84ad5 ac49ba11e983ba001d0a1c0e12.

Chapter Five: The World Is on Fire

1. Kelsey Ables, "At COP 27, an artist asks attendees to feel climate change — literally," *Washington Post*, November 12, 2022, https://www.washingtonpost .com/arts-entertainment/2022/11/12/cop-27-art-installation.

2. See "A Meditation for UN Day of Clean Air for Blue Skies," Brahma Kumaris Environment Initiative, https://eco.brahmakumaris.org/meditation-for -clean-air-blue-skies; and "Health Effects of Air Pollution," Air Pollution Impacts, Environmental Defense Fund, https://www.edf.org/health/ effects-of-air-pollution.

3. "14.9 Million Excess Deaths Associated with the COVID-19 Pandemic in 2020 and 2021," World Health Organization, May 5, 2022, https://www .who.int/news/item/05-05-2022-14.9-million-excess-deaths-were-associated -with-the-covid-19-pandemic-in-2020-and-2021.

4. "Air Pollution Linked with Higher COVID-19 Death Rates," T. H. Chan School of Public Health, Harvard University, updated May 5, 2020, https:// www.hsph.harvard.edu/news/hsph-in-the-news/air-pollution-linked-with -higher-covid-19-death-rates; and Lisa Friedman, "New Research Links Air Pollution to Higher Coronavirus Death Rates," *New York Times*, April 7, 2020, https://www.nytimes.com/2020/04/07/climate/air-pollution-coronavirus -covid.html.

5. Kate Yoder, "How Humans Kicked Off the Pyrocene, a New 'Age of Fire,'" *Grist*, November 6, 2019,https://grist.org/article/how-humans-kicked-off-the -pyrocene-a-new-age-of-fire.

6. Rosana Aguilera et al., "Wildfire Smoke Impacts Respiratory Health More Than Fine Particles from Other Sources: Observational Evidence from Southern California," *Nature Communications* 12 (March 5, 2021), https:// www. nature.com/articles/s41467-021-21708-0.

7. Jill Korsiak et al., "Long-Term Exposure to Wildfires and Cancer Incidence in Canada: A Population-Based Observational Cohort Study," *The Lancet* 6, no. 5 (May 1, 2022), https://doi.org/10.1016/S2542-5196(22)00067-5.

8. National Parks Conservation Association, "Parks Group's Report Finds 96 Percent of National Parks Are Plagued by Air Pollution," press release, May 7, 2019, https://www.npca.org/articles/2166-parks-group-s-report-finds-96 -percent-of-national-parks-are-plagued-by-air.

9. https://www.thelancet.com/journals/lanplh/article/PIIS2542 -5196(22)00090-0/fulltext See also https://www.washingtonpost.com /climate-environment/2022/05/17/pollution-caused-1-6-deaths-globally -five-straight-years-study-says/

10. "Air Pollution," World Health Organization (World Health Organization, n.d.), https://www.who.int/health-topics/air-pollution.

11. "Air Pollution," World Health Organization (World Health Organization, n.d.), https://www.who.int/health-topics/air-pollution.

12. Melissa Hogenboom, "How Air Pollution Is Doing More Than Killing Us," BBC Future (April 16, 2019), https://www.bbc.com/future/article /20190415-how-air-pollution-is-doing-more-than-killing-us.

13. Rupa Marya and Raj Patel, *Inflamed: Deep Medicine and the Anatomy of Injustice* (New York: Farrar, Straus and Giroux, 2021), 5.

14. Mary Brophy Marcus, "Pollution Kills More Than 1.7 Million Children a Year," *CBS News* (March 6, 2017) https://www.cbsnews.com/news /pollution-kills-more-than-1-7-million-children-a-year-who-reports.

15. This instructional video from the University of Michigan explains how to assemble a DIY air purifier: *Build a Do-It-Yourself Air Purifier for about $25*, YouTube (Michigan Sinus Center, 2011), https://www.youtube.com/watch ?v=kH5APw_SLUU.https://www.youtube.com/watch?v=kH5APw_SLUU.

16. "Thirty Years On, What Is the Montreal Protocol Doing to Protect the Ozone?," Chemicals & Pollution Action, UN Environment Programme, November 15, 2019, https://www.unep.org/news-and-stories/story /thirty-years-what-montreal-protocol-doing-protect-ozone.

PART II: FUNDAMENTALS OF BREATHING

Chapter Six: The Anatomy of Breathing

1. See "Anatomy Insights with Jon Zahourek," Anatomy in Clay, June 23, 2021, https://www.anatomyinclay.com/anatomy-insights-with-jon-zahourek.

Chapter Seven: Postures That Support Breath

1. *Left:* David A. Gorman, *The Body Moveable* (Etobicoke, ON: LearningMethods Publications, 2016). *Right:* Frank H. Netter, *Atlas of Human Anatomy* (Philadelphia: Elsevier, 2019).

2. "10 Fun Facts about Your Tongue and Taste Buds," OnHealth, reviewed May 14, 2021, https://www.onhealth.com/content/1/tongue_facts.

3. Jessica Wapner, "Vision and Breathing May Be the Secrets to Surviving 2020: Stanford Neurobiologist Andrew Huberman Discusses the Two Things We Can Always Control, Even during a High-Stress Election and Scary COVID Pandemic," Mental Health, *Scientific American*, November 16, 2020, https://www.scientificamerican.com/article/vision-and-breathing-may-be-the-secrets-to-surviving-2020.

Chapter Eight: The Chemistry of Respiration

1. James L. Lewis III, "Overview of Acid-Base Balance," *Merck Manual* (Consumer Version), modified September 2022, https://www.merckmanuals.com/home/hormonal-and-metabolic-disorders/acid-base-balance/overview-of-acid-base-balance#:~:text=The%20blood%20carries%20carbon%20dioxide,blood%20decreases%20(acidity%20increases).

Chapter Nine: Conversations with Breath

1. "How to Understand and Build Intimacy in Every Relationship," Healthline, reviewed April 16, 2019, https://www.healthline.com/health/intimacy#intimacy-vs-sex.

2. Mary Grace Garis and Rebecca Norris, "How Many Types of Intimacy Exist in Relationships and What Are they?," *Well + Good*, July 26, 2022, https://www.wellandgood.com/types-of-intimacy.

3. Drake Baer, "How Only Being Able to Use Logic to Make Decisions Destroyed a Man's Life," *New York Magazine* (June 14, 2016) https://www.thecut.com/2016/06/how-only-using-logic-destroyed-a-man.html.

Chapter Ten: Buteyko Breathing Education

1. Rosalba Courtney, "Healthy Breathing" in *WellBeing Magazine* (No 68 June 1997, https://buteykoclinic.com/buteyko-method/).

2. See "Buteyko Clinical Trials 1998–2017," Buteyko Clinic International, https://buteykoclinic.com/buteyko-trials.

3. See "History: The Legend of Taranaki," Taranaki Mounga, May 27, 2021, https://taranakimounga.nz/nga-mounga/history.

PART III: WORKING WITH BREATHING DISORDERS

1. Thich Nhat Hanh, *Stepping into Freedom: An Introduction to Buddhist Monastic Training* (Berkeley, CA: Parallax Press, 1997), 8.

Chapter Eleven: Dysfunctional Breathing

1.   "How to Identify and Treat Dysfunctional Breathing," Fit to Move, September 8, 2019, https://www.fittomovept.com/blog/2019/9/8/how-to-identify-and-treat-dysfunctional-breathing.

2.   Mark A Cruz, "Dysfunctional Breathing Is More Common Than You Think" (November 18, 2019, https://www.markacruzdds.com/dysfunctional-breathing-symptoms-ca/).

Chapter Twelve: Over-Breathing

1.   "Autonomic Nervous System Disorders," MedlinePlus, National Library of Medicine, https://medlineplus.gov/autonomicnervoussystemdisorders.html.

2.   "What to Know about Hyperventilation: Causes and Treatments," Healthline, updated April 29, 2019, https://www.healthline.com/health/hyperventilation.

3.   From Buteyko Breathing Education notes by Jennifer Stark.

4.   C. Gilbert, "Hyperventilation and the Body," *Accident and Emergency Nursing* 7 (1999), 130–40, https://respirasbreathing.com/documents/breathing/Hyperventilation%20and%20the%20body.pdf.

Chapter Thirteen: Asthma

1.   "Asthma Facts and Figures," Asthma and Allergy Foundation of America, updated April 2022, https://www.aafa.org/asthma-facts.

2.   "Asthma," World Health Organization, fact sheet, May 11, 2022, https://www.who.int/news-room/fact-sheets/detail/asthma.

Chapter Fourteen: Breath Holding

1.   Matt Licata, "On Therapy," from his blog *A Healing Space . . . reflections on love, meaning, and the aliveness of immediate experience* (December 11, 2020, http://alovinghealingspace.blogspot.com/2020/12/on-therapy.html)

2.   Lindsay Brownell, "Fighting Viruses Is as Easy as Breathing," Wyss Institute, Harvard University, press release, April 8, 2022, reported by Apple News, August 2022.

3.   Arlin Cuncic, "How to Develop and Practice Self-Regulation," Verywell Mind, updated January 27, 2022, https://www.verywellmind.com/how-you-can-practice-self-regulation-4163536.

Chapter Fifteen: Breathing-Disordered Sleep

1.   https://www.youtube.com/watch?v=FPgkjIvnrTQ&t=30s

2.   Matthew Walker, *Why We Sleep: Unlocking the Power of Sleep and Dreams* (New York: Scribner, 2016), 3-5.

3.   "Sleep Super Conference," (Conscious Life, 2022), https://sleepsuperconference.com.https://sleepsuperconference.com

4.   "Breathing Wellness Conference," (The Vivos Institute, 2021), https://thevivosinstitute.com/bwc22/

5. "Sleep Deprivation Disrupts Genes," Sleep Education (American Academy of Sleep Medicine, March 1, 2013), https://sleepeducation.org/sleep-deprivation-disrupts-genes.

6. Walker, *Why We Sleep*, 161.

7. Azmeh Shahid et al., "Morningness-Eveningness Questionnaire," STOP, THAT and One Hundred Other Sleep Scales, November 24, 2011, pp. 231–234, https://doi.org/10.1007/978-1-4419-9893-4_54, https://www.med.upenn.edu/cbti/assets/user-content/documents/Morningness-Eveningness%20Questionnaire.pdf

8. See María Teresa Acosta, "Sueño, memoria y aprendizaje [Sleep, memory and learning]," *Medicina* 79, Suppl. 3 (2019), https://pubmed.ncbi.nlm.nih.gov/31603840.

9. Eric J. Olson, "How Many Hours of Sleep Are Enough for Good Health?," Expert Answers, Mayo Clinic, May 15, 2021, https://www.mayoclinic.org/healthy-lifestyle/adult-health/expert-answers/how-many-hours-of-sleep-are-enough/faq-20057898.

10. Elizabeth B. Krieger, "Snooze News: What Is Sleep Dentistry?," *WebMD Magazine*, reviewed July 9, 2021, https://www.webmd.com/oral-health/features/sleep-dentistry.

11. Jay Summer, "Hypopnea," Sleep Foundation, updated October 13, 2022, https://www.sleepfoundation.org/sleep-apnea/hypopnea#:~:text=Hypopnea%20is%20a%20sleep%20breathing,like%20cardiovascular%20disease%20and%20diabetes.

12. *Sleep Med.* 2009 Aug;10(7):753-8. doi: 10.1016/j.sleep.2008.08.007. Epub 2009 Jan 30. Today, 80–85 percent goes undiagnosed.

13. Vivos Institute on LinkedIn, November 8, 2022, https://www.linkedin.com/company/vivos-institute. See also SleepSharp Editorial, "How To Know If You Have Sleep Apnea: 5 Common Signs," SleepSharp, March 8, 2020, https://www.sleepsharp.com/sleep-apnea-common-signs/#:~:text=5%20Signs%20You%20Have%20Sleep%20Apnea%20Waking%20Up,sleep%20apnea%20that%20can%20lead%20to%20anxiety%20problems.

14. Mayo Clinic staff, "Snoring," Patient Care & Health Information, Diseases & Conditions, Mayo Clinic, December 22, 2017, https://www.mayoclinic.org/diseases-conditions/snoring/symptoms-causes/syc-20377694.

15. Stef Daniel, "Snoring and the Marital Bed—It Can Ruin a Marriage," Professor's House, https://www.professorshouse.com/snoring-and-the-marital-bed.

16. See Eric Suni, "What Are the Different Types of Insomnia?," Sleep Foundation, June 24, 2022, https://www.sleepfoundation.org/insomnia/types-of-insomnia.

17. Saundra Dalton-Smith, *Sacred Rest: Recover Your Life, Renew Your Energy, Restore Your Sanity* (Nashville, TN: FathWords/Hachette, 2017).

18. Rebecca Lindsey, "Climate Change: Atmospheric Carbon Dioxide," Climate.gov, National Oceanic and Atmospheric Administration, June 23, 2022, https://www.climate.gov/news-features/understanding-climate

/climate-change-atmospheric-carbon-dioxide#:~:text=Based%20on%20 preliminary%20analysis%2C%20the,to%20the%20COVID%2D19%20 pandemic.

19. Robinson Meyer, "The Human Brain Evolved When Carbon Dioxide Was Lower," *The Atlantic*, December 20, 2019, https://www.theatlantic.com/ science/archive/2019/12/carbon-dioxide-pollution-making-people-dumber -heres-what-we-know/603826.

20. Danielle Pacheco, "The Bedroom Environment," Sleep Foundation, updated June 17, 2022, https://www.sleepfoundation.org/bedroom-environment.

21. Mayo Clinic staff, "Sleep Apnea," Patient Care & Health Information, Diseases & Conditions, Mayo Clinic, July 28, 2020, https://www.mayoclinic .org/diseases-conditions/sleep-apnea/symptoms-causes/syc-20377631.

22. Nitric oxide and humming are discussed in R. Jankowski et al., "Sinusology," *European Annals of Otorhinolaryngology, Head and Neck Diseases* 133, no. 4 (2016), https://pubmed.ncbi.nlm.nih.gov/27378676.

PART IV: TRANSFORMING YOUR WORLD AND YOUR LIFE, ONE BREATH AT A TIME

Chapter Seventeen: Breathing with Anxiety

1. Amit Ray, *Om Chanting and Meditation: A Way to Heallth and Happiness* (Rishikesh, India: Inner Light Publishers, 2010).

2. Simon Neubauer, Jean-Jacques Hublin, and Philipp Gunz, "The Evolution of Modern Human Brain Shape," *Science Advances* 4, issue 1 (January 24, 2018),https://www.science.org/doi/10.1126/sciadv.aao5961.

3. Barbara Marx Hubbard, *Conscious Evolution: Awakening the Power of Our Social Potential* (Novato, CA: New World Library, 2015), 18. Italics added.

4. Valencia Higuera, "What Is General Adaptation Syndrome?," Healthline, updated October 6, 2018, https://www.healthline.com/health/ general-adaptation-syndrome.

5. https://www.rosalbacourtney.com. See also P. R. Steffen et al., "The Impact of Resonance Frequency Breathing on Measures of Heart Rate Variability, Blood Pressure, and Mood," *Frontiers in Public Health* 5 (2017), https://www.ncbi. nlm.nih.gov/pmc/articles/PMC5575449; and "Coherent Breathing: Theory & Protocol," Coherent Breathing, Coherence LLC, https://coherentbreathing .com/theory-protocol.

6. See Claire Sissons, "What Happens When You Get an Adrenaline Rush?," *Medical News Today*, July 17, 2018, https://www.medicalnewstoday.com /articles/322490.

7. Adam Hadhazy, "Think Twice: How the Gut's 'Second Brain' Influences Mood and Well-Being," *Scientific American*, February 12, 2010, https://www.scientificamerican.com/article/gut-second-brain.

Chapter Eighteen: Awakening to Silence

1. Roche, *Radiance Sutras*, 37.

Chapter Twenty: Tying It All Together

1. Licata, Facebook Post (January 23, 2016, https://m.facebook.com/
    mattlicataphd/posts/underneath-the-narrative-of-your-life-just-below-the
    -grand-storyline-even-beneat/1503218806652001/).

Appendix C : Five-Day Buteyko Breathing Education Course

1. "Buteyko Clinic," Buteyko Clinic, April 7, 2022, https://buteykoclinic.com/.

Appendix G: Further Explorations

1. "Basketball Tip: How to Master the Jump Shot," Basketball Coach's Corner,
    U.S. Sports Camps, https://www.ussportscamps.com/tips/basketball
    /how-to-master-the-jump-shot.

2. This exploration is inspired by three sources: *Unwinding the Belly*, by Allison
    Post and Stephen Cavaliere; Susan Harper of Continuum Montage; and
    the practice of Chi Nei Tsang, a traditional Chinese massage that uses
    acupressure points in the belly to release emotions blockages and physical
    pain in order to integrate the physical, mental, emotional, and spiritual
    aspects of being.

Appendix H: Frequently Asked Questions

1. Fred Cicetti, "Here's Why You Yawn," *Live Science*, May 29, 2014, https://
    www.livescience.com/45954-the-healthy-geezer-why-do-we-yawn.html.

2. https://medlineplus.gov/ency/article/003096.htm.

3. Lindsay Dodgson, "Aaaaaaah, Really? You Would Die If You Didn't Sigh"
    Live Science (March 7, 2016) https://www.livescience.com/53953-origins-of
    -sighing-in-brain.html.

4. Mayo Clinic staff, "Bruxism (Teeth Grinding)," Patient Care & Health
    Information, Diseases & Conditions, Mayo Clinic, August 10, 2017, https://
    www.mayoclinic.org/diseases-conditions/bruxism/symptoms-causes
    /syc-20356095.

5. Lara Jansiski Motta et al., "Association between Respiratory Problems and
    Dental Caries in Children with Bruxism," *Indian Journal of Dental Research* 25,
    no. 1 (2014), https://pubmed.ncbi.nlm.nih.gov/24748291.

6. *The Dawson Academy Blog*, "The Correlation between Bruxism and Airway
    Disorders," by DeWitt Wilkerson, posted October 29, 2018, https://dental
    .thedawsonacademy.com/correlation-bruxism-airway.

7. Ann Blackford, "Chronic Throat Clearing May Be Your Body's Response
    to Irritants," University of Kentucky News, December 12, 2016,
    https://uknow.uky.edu/uk-healthcare/chronic-throat-clearing-may-be
    -your-body's-response-irritants.

8. M. Maniscalco et al., "Assessment of Nasal and Sinus Nitric Oxide Output
    Using Single-Breath Humming Exhalations," *European Respiratory Journal*
    22, no. 2 (August 2003), https://erj.ersjournals.com/content/22/2/323.
    article-info.

INDEX OF EXPLORATIONS

Chapter 20: Tying It All Together

- The End of Our Journey

Appendix G: Further Explorations

- Breathing *With*
- Being Breathed: *Sa~Ha*
- Sound Practice
- Exploring Your Tongue, Lips, and Teeth
- Feeling Support: You Have to Go Down to Go Up
- Restorative Breathing
- Befriending Your Belly

INDEX

B

ABOUT THE AUTHOR

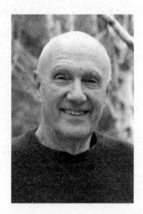

Robert Litman, creator of The Breathable Body, has been a structural integration movement teacher using Rolfing and Continuum principles for nearly 40 years. He teaches anatomy and physiology from a movement perspective and is a Buteyko Breathing educator who has guided artists, musicians, health professionals, athletes, activists, those with health challenges, retirees, and people interested in breath as a doorway to personal and spiritual growth by restoring healthy breathing rhythms, structural alignment, and coordinated, coherent movement.

Robert co-developed the Wellsprings Practitioner Program with Emilie Conrad, founder of Continuum Movement®, and co-taught with her for 18 years. He has been a faculty member and head of the departments of Anatomy and Physiology and Movement Education at the Desert Institute of the Healing Arts Massage School in Tucson, Arizona; is a certified practitioner of the Duggan/French Approach for Somatic Pattern Recognition; and is a registered educator and trainer of the Buteyko Breathing Educators Association. As a preceptor at the University of Arizona School of Integrative Medicine, Robert taught Buteyko Breathing Education principles and practice to visiting physicians for Dr. Andrew Weil. He has a graduate certification as a breathing behavior analyst at the Graduate School of Behavioral Breathing and Health Sciences in Cheyenne, Wyoming.

Robert lives on Vashon Island, Washington, and offers workshops, webinars, and private sessions in movement and breathing, locally and worldwide, including a six-month Breathable Body online training series. For information, visit thebreathablebody.com.

We hope you enjoyed this Hay House book. If you'd like to receive our online catalog featuring additional information on Hay House books and products, or if you'd like to find out more about the Hay Foundation, please contact:

Hay House, Inc., P.O. Box 5100, Carlsbad, CA 92018-5100
(760) 431-7695 or (800) 654-5126
(760) 431-6948 (fax) or (800) 650-5115 (fax)
www.hayhouse.com® • www.hayfoundation.org

———

Published in Australia by: Hay House Australia Pty. Ltd.,
18/36 Ralph St., Alexandria NSW 2015
Phone: 612-9669-4299 • *Fax:* 612-9669-4144
www.hayhouse.com.au

Published in the United Kingdom by: Hay House UK, Ltd.,
The Sixth Floor, Watson House, 54 Baker Street, London W1U 7BU
Phone: +44 (0)20 3927 7290 • *Fax:* +44 (0)20 3927 7291
www.hayhouse.co.uk

Published in India by: Hay House Publishers India,
Muskaan Complex, Plot No. 3, B-2, Vasant Kunj, New Delhi 110 070
Phone: 91-11-4176-1620 • *Fax:* 91-11-4176-1630
www.hayhouse.co.in

———

Access New Knowledge.
Anytime. Anywhere.

Learn and evolve at your own pace
with the world's leading experts.

www.hayhouseU.com

MEDITATE.
VISUALIZE.
LEARN.

Get the **Empower You**
Unlimited Audio *Mobile App*

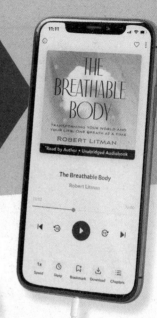

The Breathable Body
Robert Litman

Get unlimited access to the entire Hay House audio library!

You'll get:

- 500+ inspiring and life-changing **audiobooks**

- 200+ ad-free **guided meditations** for sleep, healing, relaxation, spiritual connection, and more

- Hundreds of audios **under 20 minutes** to easily fit into your day

- **Exclusive content** *only* for subscribers

- **New audios** added every week

- No credits, **no limits**

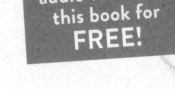

Listen to the audio version of this book for **FREE!**

★★★★★ **I ADORE this app.** I use it almost every day. Such a blessing. – Aya Lucy Rose

Scan me with your phone camera!

HAY HOUSE

TRY FOR FREE!
Go to: hayhouse.com/listen-free